# The Mechanism Of Biochemical Action Of Thyroid Hormones

## Prof. Dr. Sami A. AL- Mudhaffar

Table of Contents

Page

Page

Figures

Page

I. Abbreviations

NAD, NADH                              nicotinamide adenine dinucleotide and its reduced form.

NADP, NADPH                            nicotinamide adenine dinucleotide phosphate and its reduced form.

GSH                                    glutathione.

AMP, GMP, IMP, XMP                     the $5'$-phosphates of the ribonucleosides of adenine, guanine, hypoxanthine and xanthine.

ADP                                    the 5(pyro)-diphosphate of adenosine.

ATP                                    the 5(pyro)-triphosphate of adenosine.

RNA, DNA                               ribonucleic acid, deoxyribonucleic acid.

Pi, PPi                                orthophosphate and pyrophosphate.

Tris                                   tris(hydroxymethyl) aminomethane.

EDTA                                   ethylenediamine tetraacetate.

BMR                                    basal metabolic rate.

$L-T_3$                                $3, 5, 3'$-triiodo-L-thyronine.

$L-T_4$                                $3, 5, 3', 5'$-tetraiodo-L-thyronine.

$D-T_4$                                $3, 5, 3', 5'$-tetraiodo-D-thyronine.

$L-T_4$ acetic acid                    $3, 5, 3', 5'$-tetraiodo thyroacetic acid.

L-T$_3$ acetic acid                    3, 5, 3'-triiodothyroacetic acid

L-T$_4$ propionic acid             3, 5, 3', 5'-tetraiodothyropropionic acid

L-T$_3$ propionic acid             3, 5, 3'-triiodothyropropionic acid

L-T$_2$ thyronine                       3, 5-diiodo-L-thyronine.

L-T$_2$ tyrosine                         3, 5-diiodo-L-tyrosine

L-T$_2$ propionic acid             3, 5-diiodothyropropionic acid

## II. Introduction and Literature Review

In 1657, Thomas Wharton, gave the name glandula thyreiodea to the thyroid gland (1). Sir Charles Harington (2) has reviewed the historical background of the thyroid gland and he pointed out that the Chinese used seaweed preparations as a remedy for goitre. Courtois (3) in 1813, discovered the element iodine in saltpetre. FayFe (4) found iodine in the sponge. Coindet (5) cured goitrous patients with burnt sponge and potassium iodide. This led to the concept that goitre may be due to an iodine deficiency. The successful treatment of goitre by burnt sponge and of thyroid administration led Kocher in 1883 (6) to suggest that the thyroid gland might itself contain iodine. In 1895, Baumann (7) reported that the thyroid gland contains iodine in a protein fraction, which on hydrolysis yielded a substance called by him "iodothrin." This helped Kendall (8) to isolate a crystalline, physiologically active product which contained 65% iodine. He named it thyroxine. The structure of thyroxine was established by Harington (9). The combination of labelling of iodinated compounds and chromatographic separation has revealed many compounds which are present in the thyroid gland in amounts too small to detect by other methods. The results of this combined approach was the identification of the thyroid hormone $L-T_3$ by Gross and Pitt-Rivers in 1952 (10).

In spite of the enormous amount of work that has been done in connection with thyroid gland and its hormones, the mechanism of action of thyroid hormones has not yet been elucidated. Understanding the mechanism of action of any hormone is complicated by:

1. Tissues respond to more than one hormone, additively, permissively or antagonistically.

2. Each hormone exhibits multiple effects.

3. The observed response is dependent on the dose. The dependence on the dose is well illustrated in the case of thyroid hormones and to lesser extent by other hormones. In warm-blooded animals, small amounts of thyroxine have anabolic effects, but large doses exert a catabolic effect (11).

4. Tissue specificity and sites of action. For some time, it was believed that each hormone acted on a specific "target" organ. However, the evidence is not clear-cut and this concept is no longer considered seriously. For example, almost all animal tissue respond to thyroid hormones and the response is varied.

In vivo, thyroid hormones alter respiration, temperature regulation, growth, development, response to other hormones, nerve function and they modify the metabolism of proteins, fats, carbohy-

drates, nucleic acids, vitamins, anions, and cations. With this
knowledge, the question arises whether one or more of the multiple
biological actions can be directly attributed to a primary effect at
the cell level or whether they represent only a secondary or remote
manifestation of the primary interaction. So far there has been no
success in classification of the primary and secondary biological
effects. Nevertheless, any explanation of how thyroid hormones act,
must take these varied biological effects into account. But, before
evaluating these actions we must discuss those actions which are known
in some detail.

1. Anabolic effects with respect to protein and lipid
metabolism.

2. The regulation of basal metabolic rate.

3. Growth and Development.

1. Anabolic effects with respect to protein and lipid
metabolism. The absence or excess of thyroid hormones causes
qualitative and quantitative changes in almost every body constituent.
These have been covered by a voluminous literature since the
beginning of the century (12-14). Hypothyroid subjects have a lower
capacity to synthesize protein than do euthyroid subjects which upon
thyroid hormone administration is restored to normal. However,
administration of the same dose of $L-T_3$ to normal subjects decreases

the rate of protein synthesis.

Thyroid hormones influence the metabolism of lipids. The administration of thyroid hormone to hypothyroid patients results in an increase in serum lipids, but in the hyperthyroid state the serum lipid level is below normal (15).

The influence of thyroid hormones on lipid and protein metabolism appears to be more profound than on the metabolism of carbohydrates, water, electrolytes, vitamins, and coenzymes. Most people think that the effect on the latter constituents is a secondary action to the effect on protein. The effect on carbohydrate metabolism is not clear and often contradictory. But it is , however, agreed that thyroid hormones have an overall glycogenolytic effect (16-18).

2. Regulation of B. M. R. Regulation of BMR is the best known of the biological actions of thyroid hormones. Most workers think the calorigenic action is the fundamental property of the thyroid hormone and that other biological actions are secondary to it. This is based on the fact that thyroid hormones appear to control some enzymes involved in mitochondrial oxidative phosphorylation, which are directly tied with the basal metabolic rate. Some investigators consider that an increase in respiration is a result of the uncoupling of oxidative phosphorylation by these hormones; or due to swelling of the mitochondria. Those hypotheses which may explain the calorigenic

action have not been successful in explaining the multiple biological actions of thyroid hormones, although some of these may explain the toxic effect of the hormones.

3. Growth and Development. Thyroid hormones accelerate growth, maturation of special tissues, and the acceleration of amphibian metamorphosis. The best example which illustrates the effect of thyroid hormones on general body growth is dwarfism, which is associated with hypothyroidism at early stages in life. This abnormality can be corrected by administration of thyroid hormones (19-20).

The growth effect has not received the same attention as has the calorigenic action. This comes from two reasons:

a. Growth is less susceptible to study than is the B.M.R.

b. Growth promoting effect of thyroid hormones becomes progressively diminished with the age of the animal.

The role of thyroid hormones in development is well illustrated in amphibian metamorphosis (21). Many reviews on the role of thyroid hormones in amphibian metamorphosis are available (22). Induction or acceleration of metamorphosis in the frog by thyroid hormones is perhaps the most sensitive of all biological assays for comparing the potencies of substances with thyroid hormone like action (23).

Although the major physiological responses to the thyroid hormones are well known, a mechanism by which these hormones bring about these actions is still not known.

In spite of the voluminous work on the subject, no single concept broad enough to explain the multiple actions of these hormones has been produced.

A number of hypotheses have been proposed. Earlier suggestions on the mode of action of the thyroid hormones included:

a. Making the tissue more responsive to nervous stimulations (24).

b. Control of vitamin balance (13).

c. An interaction with other hormones (13).

d. Direct interaction between hormones and enzymes. This hypothesis is the most favored. The effect of thyroid hormones on the activity of many enzymes has been tested, but the physiological significance of these responses has been difficult to assess.

Direct interaction studies have lacked hormonal specificity. For example, $D-T_4$, which is biologically inactive, is as potent as the natural L-isomer in activating mitochondrial ATPase (25). The response of many enzymes to thyroid hormones was observed at a concentration that would be considered pharmacological rather than a physiological (26).

e. Interaction of thyroid hormones with mitochondrial membranes. This effect has received considerable attention, but the results have been inconsistent and the physiological significance has been difficult to determine.

For example Tapley (27) and Tapley et al. (28) reported that a concentration of $L-T_4$ of the order of $10^{-5}M$ caused mitochondria to swell very rapidly. $L-T_3$ was about as active as $L-T_4$ in causing liver mitochondria to swell, whereas the deaminated derivatives which have a relatively low $L-T_4$ -like activity in the whole animal, also had a strong effect on liver mitochondrial stability in vitro. He found that D-isomers of $T_3$ and T4 were as effective as the L-isomers. He concluded that the uncoupling of oxidative phosphorylation in mitochondria by $L-T_4$ was not due to its direct interaction with any of the various enzymes involved in oxidative phosphorylation, but rather due to the hormonal effect on the mitochondrial structure. It should be mentioned that iodine and iodine cyanide (ICN) can cause swelling of liver mitochondria (29) (30).

Since numerous compounds which have no hormonal activity in vivo and since $L-T_3$ is equally as effective as $D-T_4$, it does not seem likely that swelling of the mitochondria is the site of action of thyroid hormones.

f. Uncoupling of oxidative phosphorylation. In 1952, Lardy and Wellman reported that cellular respiration and metabolism can be effectively controlled by uncoupling of phosphorylation from oxidation (31). Lardy and Maley (25) and Klemperer (32) found that $L-T_4$, and $L-T_3$ added to isolated liver mitochondria uncoupled oxidative phosphorylation. However, the effect was observed only when high doses of hormone were administered. No uncoupling, or loss of respiratory control was observed with small amounts of hormones (20ug/100g of body weight). However, 1700ug/100g of body weight lowered the P:O ratio (11). Other workers (33) have reported that under conditions in which L-T4, added in vitro to normal mitochondria, did not influence oxidative phosphorylation, but the addition of $L-T_4$ to liver mitochondria, from thyroidectomized rats increased succinate oxidation significantly without reducing the efficiency of the associated phosphorylation. These data suggested that thyroid hormones have an indirect effect on oxidative phosphorylation.

g. Control of Nucleic acid synthesis. Thyroid hormones stimulate protein synthesis. It is becoming apparent that the regulation of protein and nucleic acid synthesis may be an important area of hormone action. Studies using labe led amino acids show that administration of thyroid hormones stimulates the rate of protein synthesis in vivo and in cell-free systems. DuToit (34) found that the incorporation of radioactive alanine into protein by liver slices was depressed after thyroidectomy and was stimulated after large doses of thyroxine. DuToit was the first to show accelerated incorporation of labeled amino acids into protein. Little attention had been paid to this until Sokoloff undertook his studies on protein synthesis.

Sokoloff and Kaufman (35) in 1959, tested the effect of $10^{-5}$M L-$T_4$ on the in vitro incorporation of DL-leucine-1-$^{14}$C into the protein of rat liver homogenates. They found an increase in the rate of amino acid incorporation and suggested that the acceleration of metabolic rate characteristic of L-$T_4$ action may be secondary to the stimulation of energy requiring reactions such as protein synthesis. In 1960 the same workers (36) found that L-$T_4$ at 100ug/100g of body weight for 10 days stimulated amino acid incorporation in vivo and in vitro. The increase in protein synthetic activity in the L-$T_4$ pretreated rats was found to be associated with the mitochondrial fraction. The L-$T_4$ effect in vitro was dependent on the presence of mitochondria and a substrate for oxidative phosphorylation. The effect was not observed when the oxidative phosphorylation system was replaced by a creatine phosphate-ATP generating system. Although mitochondria were essential for the L-$T_4$ stimulation, the actual effect was to accelerate the amino acid incorporation into protein of the microsomal sub fractions. D-$T_4$ when added in vitro directly to the cell homogenates was as effective as L-$T_4$. L-$T_3$ was effective when administered in vivo but had very low activity when added in vitro. Sokoloff et al. (37) later presented evidence that the step involving the transfer of aminoacyl RNA to a microsomal protein, was the step stimulated by L-T4. The stimulation of this step required the mitochondria. Weiss and Sokoloff later found (38) that L-thyroxine increases the in vivo incorporation of radioactive amino acids into protein of liver, kidney, and heart but not of spleen, testes, or brain. Then in 1964, Sokoloff et al. (39) reported the stimulation of amino acid incorporation into protein was independent of RNA synthesis. They noted that inhibition of DNA-dependent RNA polymerase by actinomycinD and DNase has no effect on the rate of amino acid incorporation into protein or the response to thyroxine. Stein and Gross (40) and Hanson et al. (42) were unable to repeat Sokoloff's experiment. Roodyn et al. (42) found that mitochondrial and microsomal amino acid incorporation are independent processes.

A stimulation of protein synthesis by thyroid hormones was observed by Frieden (43) during amphibian metamorphosis. He found a rapid appearance of urea cycle enzymes, adult hemoglobin, serum albumin, and other liver and tail enzymes such as dehydro-genases, phosphatases and ribonuclease (44). Herner and Frieden (45) have established that there occurs beside stimulation of protein synthesis, an increase in the turnover of RNA in the liver. They suggested that the thyroid hormones regulate the metabolism of nucleic acid.

A series of experiments by Tata and coworkers (46-49) opened the door to a new approach in solving the problem of the mode of action of thyroid hormones. They established that the sequence of events following the injection of a single, small dose of $L-T_3$(10ug/ 100 g body weight) into a rat was an increase in the specific activity of rapidly labeled nuclear RNA beginning at 3-4 hours after hormone administration followed at 7 hours by a stimulation of RNA polymerase. A rise in the ribosomal RNA started at 12 hours and at 18 hours protein synthesis was stimulated.

Necheles (50) found that at $10^{-7}$M of $L-T_4$ purine biosynthesis was increased and he suggested that thyroid hormones may not act directly on the nucleic acid themselves but rather by somehow controlling the availability of purine nucleotides for RNA synthesis.

It was reported that thyroid hormones stimulated the incorporation of glycine-1-$^{14}$C into the purines of the soluble fraction of livers from growth-arrested, sulfaguanidine-fed rats (68). The purines were isolated after incubation and the distribution of $^{14}$C in the purines and the concentrations of the purines suggested that the reaction stimulated by thyroid hormones was IMP to AMP. At that time it also appeared that the concentration of guanine decreased. Further work confirmed that the in vitro addition of thyroid hormones to a soluble fraction of rat liver stimulated the conversion of IMP to AMP. The optimum concentration of $T_3$ and $T_4$ was $2.5 \times 10^{-9}$M, and $2.5 \times 10^{-5}$M respectively. Higher concentrations were less effective. The decrease in the concentration of guanine suggested that thyroid hormones also appeared to inhibit the synthesis of GMP.

Since thyroid hormones stimulated the conversion of IMP to AMP (52) and, IMP is also a precursor of GMP, it appeared possible that thyroid hormones inhibited one of the two reactions involved in the conversion of IMP to GMP. However, the inhibition of GMP synthesis may be more apparent than real because the stimulation of AMP synthesis may decrease the availability of IMP for GMP synthesis. It was the purpose of this dissertation to investigate the effect of thyroid hormones on GMP synthesis. The following scheme illustrates the relationship of IMP to both AMP and GMP.

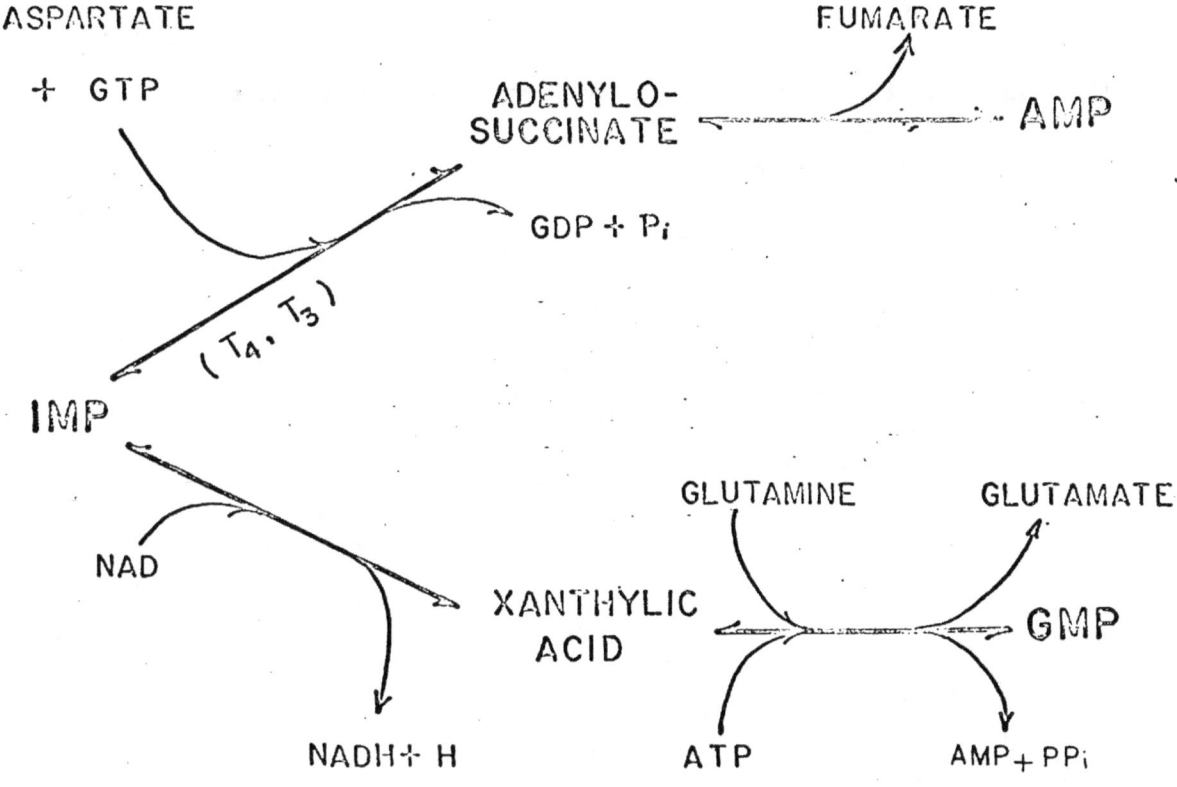

III.  The inhibition of inosine monophosphate-dehydrogenase by

thyroid hormones in vitro.

## Introduction

While investigating the incorporation of glycine-l-$^{14}$C into the purines of the soluble fraction of rat liver, Mah and Ackerman noted that the addition of thyroid hormones stimulated the synthesis of AMP but appeared to inhibit the synthesis of GMP (51). It was established later that L-T$_4$ and L-T$_3$ stimulated the conversion of IMP to AMP (52). Since IMP is a precursor of both AMP and GMP it was of interest to determine whether the apparent inhibition of GMP synthesis by thyroid hormones was due to a direct inhibition of one or more of the enzymes in the pathway leading to GMP or whether stimulation of AMP synthesis decreased the availability of IMP for GMP synthesis.

IMP has been established as a precursor of purine nucleo-tides by the work of Greenberg (53) and Buchanan and Schulman (54). Magasanik and coworkers (55) (56), Abrams and Bently (57), and Lagerkvist (58)(59) have studied the conversion of IMP to GMP in bacterial, mammalian, and avian systems, respectively. The first reaction involved in the enzymic conversion of IMP to XMP was demonstrated in a soluble extract from rabbit bone marrow by

Abrams and Bently (60), in E. coli extracts, by Gehring and
Magasanik (61) and by Turner and King in pea seeds (62). In these
systems the initial enzymatic step is the oxidation of IMP by the NAD
linked enzyme, IMP-dehydrogenase. The second step involves the
conversion of XMP to yield GMP and this reaction requires ATP and
glutamine or ammonium ions (65).

The two reactions proceed as follows:

(1)　$\text{IMP} \xrightarrow[\text{NADH} + \text{H}]{\text{NAD}} \text{XMP}$

(2)　$\text{XMP} + \text{ATP} + \text{glutamine} \xrightarrow{\text{Mg}} \text{GMP} + \text{Glutamate} + \text{AMP} + \text{PPi}$

This investigation is concerned with the isolation of IMP-
dehydrogenase from rat liver and the effect of thyroid hormones on
this enzyme.

## Experimental Procedure

### Materials and Methods

IMP was purchased from Sigma Chemical Co., ATP and NAD from P-L Biochemicals, Inc. $L-T_4$, purchased from Sigma Chemical Co., was recrystallized from $Na_2CO_3$ and ethanol, mp 232-234C (66). $L-T_3$, purchased from Sigma Chemical Co., was recrystallized from boiling 2N HCL, mp 201-203C (67). $D-T_4$ was purchased from K & K Laboratories. $L-T_4$ propionic acid, $L-T_4$ acetic acid, $L-T_3$ propionic acid, $T_2$-propionic acid and $T_2$-tyrosine were purchased from Cyclo Chemical Corp. These compounds were used without further purification. $L-T_3$ and $L-T_4$ and derivatives of these were dissolved in 0.05 ml of 2N NaOH and diluted to appropriate volumes with 0.02M tris-phosphate buffer, pH 8.3.

Only male, Sprague-Dawley rats between 8-9 weeks of age were used for these experiments. Thyroid hormone-depleted rats were animals that had been fed a complete diet containing 1% of sulfaguanidine for a period of 5 to 6 weeks. Such rats gain less than 2 grams per week and weigh 120-145 grams when 9 weeks of age(68).

Crude preparations of IMP-dehydrogenase were made from the livers of thyroid hormone depleted rats. The livers from 2-5 of such rats were pooled and homogenized with 2.5 volumes (w/v) of cold $(5^\circ) 10^{-3}$M EDTA for 30 seconds with a Sorvall Omni-mixer at one-half maximal speed. The homogenate was centrifuged at 100,000 x g for 1 hour. The supernatant fraction was dialyzed against 2 liters of water for 20 hrs. with 3 changes of water. The dialyzed preparation was used for some enzyme assays. An acetone powder was prepared, as will be described, and used for studies of GMP synthesis. For later experiments, a partially purified enzyme was prepared as follows:

Purification of IMP-dehydrogenase: All of the purification steps were carried out at $0-3^\circ$ except where noted:

(1) Preparation of acetone powder. Male Sprague-Dawley rats, sulfaguanidine-fed, or normal rats (150-180 g), were sacrified by decapitation, the livers were removed, rinsed with $10^{-3}$M EDTA, chilled in ice, weighed and homogenized in 2.5 volumes (w/v) of cold $10^{-3}$M EDTA. The homogenate was centrifuged at 100,000 x g for one hour in a Spinco Model L centrifuge. Seven to eight volumes of cold $(-11^\circ)$ acetone were added slowly with stirring. The resulting slurry was stirred for several minutes. The precipitate was collected on a Buchner funnel and washed twice with acetone, twice with ether,

and immediately dried over phosphorous pentoxide in a desiccator with solid paraffin to absorb the ether. The acetone powder could be stored at -10°c for about 10 days without loss of activity.

(2) Ammonium sulfate fractionation. The liver acetone powder (1-2 gms) was extracted with 15 volumes (w/v) of 0.05 M tris-phosphate buffer pH 8.3 for 30 minutes at 5° and centrifuged at 13,000 x g for 60 minutes. The enzyme was precipitated from the supernatant solution by the addition of $(NH_4)_2SO_4$ until a concentration equivalent to 30-40% of saturation was achieved. The precipitate was dissolved in 5.0 ml of the tris-phosphate buffer containing 60 mg of cysteine-HCL.

(3) DEAE Sephadex A-50 Column. The redissolved precipitate was applied to a DEAE Sephadex A-50 column (10 x 1.5 cm$^2$) previously equilibrated with the same buffer and containing 0.2 u moles of 2 -mercaptoethanol per ml. The enzyme was eluted from the column with an increasing concentration gradient (69) of buffer (300 ml of 0.5 M tris-phosphate, pH 8.3 in the reservoir added to 100 ml of 0.05 M buffer in the mixing chamber). Five milliliter fractions were collected. The first 5 ml were discarded and the next 5 ml contained approximately 60% of the recoverable enzyme activity. This fraction was used for enzyme assays. Solutions of this enzyme at 5° lost 50% of their activity in 24 hours.

Initially only livers from growth-arrested, sulfaguanidine-fed rats were used as a source of the enzyme because thyroid hormones had no effect when the enzyme was prepared from livers of normal rats, nor did these enzyme preparations respond to the thyroid hormones after passage through neutral Sephadex G-50. Presumably, the enzyme from normal rats was saturated with tightly bound thyroid hormones but, after passage through DEAE Sephadex, a satisfactory enzyme preparation was obtained.

Crude enzyme from brains and testes were prepared as follows: Rat brain or testes were homogenized with 2.5 volumes (w/v) of 0.05 M tris-phosphate buffer and then centrifuged at 100,000 x g for 1 hour. The supernatant fraction was used for the enzyme assays.

Enzyme Assays

(1) Assay for GMP synthesis: This method is a modification of the method used by Abrams and Bently (57) and depends upon the fact that the absorbancy of GMP in acid at 290 mu is 30 times that of IMP. After incubation, 0.2 ml of 3.6 M perchloric acid were added. The precipitated protein was centrifuged out, and absorption of the supernatant was measured at 290 mu with a Beckman DU Spectrophotometer against a reference cuvette which contained the supernatant fraction from a reaction vessel that had been incubated

with all ingredients except IMP. IMP was added after the addition of perchloric acid.

(2) Assay for XMP synthesis: All assays of IMP dehydrogenase were followed by measuring the reduction of NAD at 340 mu in a Beckman Model DU Spectrophotometer against blank without enzyme. One unit of enzyme activity is defined as the synthesis of one mu mole of reduced NAD (NADH) per minute at 28°. NADH was calculated from its molar absorbancy index of $6.2 \times 10^3$ (70).

Protein was estimated by the spectrophotometric method of Warburg and Christian (71).

## Results

Purification of IMP dehydrogenase: Table I shows the results of the purification of IMP dehydrogenase. A 34-fold purification was achieved based on the activity of acetone powder.

Effect of pH: The activity of the enzyme was studied in a series of buffers containing 0.05 M tris-phosphate and over the pH range 7.5---9.0. The pH-activity curve (Figure 1) showed a sharp optimum at approximately pH 8.3 . The optimum pH for this enzyme from pea-seed has been reported to be 8.0 (62).

Specificity of the IMP dehydrogenase: Fig. 2 shows that NAD is more effective as a cofactor for IMP-dehydrogenase than NADP. When NADP was substituted for NAD at the same concentration, the

the reaction was only 70% of that obtained with NAD.

The effect of thyroid hormones: Fig. 3 illustrates that L-T$_3$ at $10^{-9}$M inhibited GMP synthesis throughout a 24 min. reaction period. Fig. 4 illustrates the inhibition of IMP dehydrogenase by L-T$_3$ at $10^{-9}$M in crude preparations. Both L-T$_4$ and L-T$_3$ inhibited IMP dehydrogenase (Figs. 5, 6) but the degree of inhibition was dependent upon the concentration of the hormones. The maximum inhibitory effect occurred with $10^{-7}$M of L-T$_4$, but increasing the concentration to $10^{-5}$M resulted in little or no inhibition. Similar results were observed with L-T$_3$, except that the maximum inhibitory effect occurred with $10^{-9}$M of L-T$_3$, and again, increasing the concentration decreased the inhibitory effect. This phenomenon, or "peak" effect was also observed during the investigation of AMP synthesis. It was observed that the stimulation of AMP synthesis was maximal with $10^{-9}$M of L-T$_3$ or $10^{-5}$M of L-T$_4$, but as the concentration of these hormones was increased, the stimulatory effect decreased(52).

Fig. 7 shows that D-T$_4$, which is inactive as a thyroid hormone, was also ineffective as an inhibitor of IMP dehydrogenase. It stimulated the reaction when its concentration was $10^{-6}$M or higher.

To establish that the synthesis of XMP, the product of IMP oxidation was inhibited by thyroid hormones, the purified enzyme preparation was incubated with L-T$_4$ ($10^{-7}$M) or L-T$_3$ ($10^{-9}$M) as described under Table 2 and after incubation, the reaction mixture was heated with HCL to hydrolyze the nucleotides (57). One-half milliliter of each hydrolysate was chromatographed on filter paper (S and S 589, green lable) with 95% ethanol: 1.0 M $NH_4$-acetate pH 7.5(7:3). Authentic xanthine was developed on a separate chromatogram and also, 0.1 umole of xanthine were cochromatographed with 0.5 ml of the hydrolysate from the control reaction. The $R_f$ of xanthine was 0.42. Those spots having an $R_f$ of 0.42 on each chromatogram were eluted with 0.3 M tris-phosphate buffer, pH 7.6, which was then adjusted to pH 10 with KOH and centrifuged. The absorption specturm of the alkaline solutions was measured, and measured again after the solutions were made acid by the addition of HCL. These measurements were made against an extract of section $R_f$ 0.42 from a blank paper chromatogram developed with the same solvent system. The concentration of xanthine was calculated from its molar absorbancy index ($9.3 \times 10^3$) (70) at 276 mu at pH 10.

The spectral data are summarized in Table 2. The data of xanthine isolated from the reaction vessels agrees with the data for xanthine that has been co-chromatographed with the hydrolysate from the control reaction. The quantity of xanthine recovered from the reaction vessels demonstrates again the inhibition of IMP-dehydrogenase by $L-T_3$ and $L-T_4$.

Fig. 13 shows $L-T_3$ propionic acid, which is physiologically active, was also effective as an inhibitor of IMP dehydrogenase. It inhibited the reaction at $10^{-5}$M maximally.

Fig. 14 shows $L-T_3$ propionic acid, which is also physiologically active, was effective as an inhibitor of IMP dehydrogenase. It inhibited the reaction maximally at $10^{-5}$M and to lesser extent by $10^{-7}$M and $10^{-9}$M.

Table 4 shows neither $L-T_4$ nor $L-T_3$ inhibited the reduction of NAD by brain although a slight inhibition of the testes system was noted.

Fig. 8 shows that when $10^{-9}$M of L-T$_3$ was incubated simultaneously with $10^{-7}$M of L-T$_4$, the inhibitory effect was greater than that due to either alone. But if the concentration of L-T$_4$ was increased to $10^{-5}$M, the inhibitory effect appeared to be due to L-T$_3$ alone. This is consistant with the data shown in Fig. 6 and Fig. 7 where the effect of $10^{-5}$M of L-T$_4$ was negligible.

The effect of thyronine analogues on IMP-dehydrogenase: Fig. 9 shows that T$_2$-tyrosine, which is inactive as a thyroid hormone, was also ineffective as an inhibitor of IMP dehydrogenase. It stimulated the reaction when its concentration was $10^{-7}$M or higher. The stimulatory effect was a peak when the concentration of the compound was $10^{-7}$M.

In Fig. 10 T$_2$-propionic acid, which is inactive as a thyroid hormone, was also ineffective as an inhibitor of IMP-dehydrogenase. Slight inhibition was observed with $10^{-7}$M and $10^{-9}$M but $10^{-5}$M stimulated the reaction in a manner similar to D-T$_4$.

Fig. 11 illustrates T$_2$-thyronine, which is inactive as thyroid hormones, was also ineffective as an inhibitor of IMP dehydrogenase. It stimulated the reaction when its concentration was $10^{-9}$M to $10^{-5}$M.

Fig. 12 shows that L-T$_4$ acetic acid, which is active as a thyroid hormone, was an effective inhibitor of IMP dehydrogenase. It inhibited the reaction at $10^{-5}$M maximally.

## Discussion

The results in the preceeding section have demonstrated that thyroid hormones inhibit IMP dehydrogenase. The inhibition by both $L-T_4$ and $L-T_3$ was biphasic and the same phenomena was observed in the studies on the synthesis of AMP (52). Other workers have also noted biphasic effects of thyroid hormones on other systems. Necheles (50) observed a peak stimulatory effect on protein synthesis when $L-T_4$ was added to rabbit bone marrow slices. A slight increase or decrease in the concentration of $L-T_4$ above or below $10^{-7}M$ caused a drastic decrease in the stimulatory effect. Malic dehydrogenase is inhibited by $10^{-5}M$ of $L-T_4$ and stimulated by $10^{-6}M$ (72-74). $L-T_4$ at $10^{-5}M$ caused a three to five-fold increase in benzoyl aspartate production of segments of pea epicotyls excised from the apex of the third internode. With $10^{-6}M$, the stimulatory effect decreased (75). Sugisawa (76), observed that $7 \times 10^{-7}M$ of $L-T_4$ stimulated liver succinic dehydrogenase, but $1.4 \times 10^{-6}M$ inhibited this enzyme. $L-T_4$ and $L-T_3$ stimulate ascorbic acid oxidase at low concentration and inhibit it at high concentration (77). The biphasic effect is also observed in intact animals and in isolated tissue systems. It has been known for a long time that, whereas small doses of thyroid hormones promote body growth, large amounts will arrest growth or even cause a substantial weight loss (78) (79). Similarly, the anabolic effects of thyroid hormones on protein and lipid metabolism and on glycolysis at near physiological level can be reversed with larger or pharmacological doses (80). A similar biphasic effect has also been demonstrated in vitro in the growth of cultured embryonic chick limb-bone rudiments (81). Many observations would suggest that the biphasic effect is one of the features of these hormones. Further kinetics studies are necessary to understand the biphasic effect of $L-T_3$ and $L-T_4$ on adenylosuccinate synthetase and IMP-dehydrogenase and whether or not the effect on these two enzymes explains the biphasic response of the intact animal.

The results shown in Fig. 8 suggests that $L-T_3$ and $L-T_4$ act independently on IMP-dehydrogenase since $10^{-9}M$ $L-T_3$ with $10^{-7}M$ $L-T_4$ enhanced the inhibition. If the concentration of $L-T_4$ was increased to $10^{-5}M$, the inhibitory effect decreased. Such synergism of both $L-T_3$ and $L-T_4$ at their optimum concentration seem to require at least two sites, one for $L-T_3$ and other for $L-T_4$ on the protein molecule, and the pattern of interaction suggests that one is specific for $L-T_3$ and the other for $L-T_4$. Similar results were found when both hormones were incubated simultaneously with adenylosuccinate synthetase (65).

Initially only livers from growth-arrested sulfaguanidine fed rats were used as a source of the enzyme because thyroid hormones had no effect when the enzyme was prepared from livers of normal rats, nor did enzyme preparation from normal rats respond to thyroid hormones after passage through neutral Sephadex G-50. Presumably, the enzyme from normal rats was saturated with tightly bound thyroid hormones but after passage through DEAE Sephadex the hormones were separated from the enzyme. This is consistent with reports in which Sephadex is used to separate protein bound hormone from free hormone of plasma (114, 82). The protein bound fraction is eluted from the column unchanged. The same problem was encounted during the purification of adenylosuccinate synthetase(65).

D-$T_4$, $T_2$ tyrosine, $T_2$ propionic acid and $T_2$ thyronine are ineffective as an inhibitor of IMP dehydrogenase. These compounds are inactive as thyroid hormones, i.e. they do not promote the growth of thyroidectomized animals and have no or slight activity in stimulating the BMR (82) (83).

L-$T_4$ acetic acid, L-$T_4$ propionic acid and L-$T_3$ propionic acid, inhibit IMP dehydrogenase. These compounds are physiologically active (82, 83). They have been shown to raise the metabolic rate of thyroidectomized rats (84), stimulate oxygen consumption and increase body temperature. Also, they are very potent in promoting metamorphosis of the tadpole and are effective anti-goitrogenic agents(13).

The effect of the above compounds on IMP dehydrogenase shows a relationship between their activity and chemical structure. The diphenyl ether grouping is essential for activity since diiodotyrosine is inert. Thyronine derivatives must contain at least three halogen substituents. An alanine side chain is important but substitution by other aliphatic acids will increase their activity. However, no maxima were observed in the concentration range tested which contrasts with the effect of $L-T_3$ and $L-T_4$. Thyroid hormones are ineffective as inhibitors of IMP dehydrogenase of rat brain and rat testes. Respiration of brain and testes tissues from adult animals does not respond to thyroid hormone status (13) (85). Others have found that thyroxine stimulates amino acid incorporation in the testes, but brain is not effected by thyroid hormones (38). The activity of IMP dehydrogenase in both tissue was independent of the concentration of the enzyme used. The activity of the enzyme was higher when it was diluted than when it was concentrated. This suggests the possibility that an inhibitor was associated with the enzyme and it was diluted out when the lower enzyme concentration was used, or that the observed reduction of NAD was not due to IMP dehydrogenase.

This investigation provides an explanation for the decreased incorporation of glycine $1-^{14}C$ into guanine when $L-T_3$ and $L-T_4$ were added to the supernatant fraction of rat liver (51).

The effect of thyroid hormones on IMP dehydrogenase is physiologically meaningful since it is well correlated with reported in vivo effects of the hormones. Both $L-T_3$ and $L-T_4$ inhibit the reaction at concentrations which may be considered physiological and $L-T_3$ is more effective as an inhibitor than is $L-T_4$. Also the compounds which are inactive in vivo are ineffective as inhibitors of IMP dehydrogenase and those which are active in vivo are potent inhibitors. Furthermore, the hormones do not inhibit IMP dehydrogenase from rat brain and testis.

These results and the importance of this enzyme in nucleic aicd metabolism, fits the concept of a site of action for thyroid hormones better than many previous suggestions, but the significance of an inhibition of GMP synthesis is not clear. It may be that GMP, GDP, or GTP functions as an effector of some key enzyme in RNA synthesis or protein synthesis and this control will be limited if thyroid hormones are absent. Others (65) have found that thyroid hormones stimulate AMP synthesis, specifically adenylosuccinate synthetase. Since IMP is the common precursor for both AMP and GMP, these results become important because they indicate that this

branched pathway is subject to the control of thyroid hormones.
Therefore thyroid hormones control the cellular AMP/GMP ratio
by stimulating AMP synthesis concomitant with an inhibition of GMP
synthesis. Thus, this new hypothesis for the control of metabolism
by thyroid hormones is proposed. Some additional experiments
were run in an effort to establish the significance of the effect of
thyroid hormones on AMP and GMP synthesis. These are exploratory
in nature and are presented in the following sections.

IV.  The effect of thyroid hormones on AMP synthesis in brain

and testes in vitro.

## Introduction

That the site of action of thyroid hormones is adenylosuccinate synthetase and IMP dehydrogenase is strongly supported by several lines of evidence. Both enzymes are effected maximally by concentrations of the hormones which may be considered physiological. Stimulation of AMP synthesis by thyroid hormones (65) is correlated with the concept that thyroid hormones regulate energy metabolism since AMP is a precursor of ATP. Also, analogues of the hormones effect a response on these two enzymes that is correlated with their physiological effects, i.e. those which are inactive in vivo, have no effects on the enzyme whereas those which are effective in vivo are also effective in vitro. In addition, it was noted in the previous section, that IMP dehydrogenase of rat brain and testes were not inhibited by either thyroxine or triiodothyronine. This is significant because neither rat brain nor testes respond to thyroid hormone status (13). It was reported that the administration of large doses of thyroxine to rats stimulated respiration of liver, kidney, heart, skeletal muscle, and but had no effect on the respiration of testes. It is known (85) that thyroidectomy has little or no effect on respiration of rat brain or testes whereas the respiration of other tissues falls rapidly to levels characteristics of the hypothyroid condition. Therefore, if the site of action of thyroid hormones is considered to be adenylosuccinate synthetase and IMP-dehydrogenase, then it may be expected that these enzymes are absent in brain and testes, or, they are insensitive to thyroid hormones. The effect of thyroid hormones on adenylosuccinate synthetase had not been tested, in brain and testes and therefore it was desirable to test the effect of thyroid hormones on this enzyme in these tissues. No response to thyroid hormones would provide additional support to the hypothesis that the site of action of thyroid hormones in adenylosuccinate synthetase. It is the purpose of these experiments to provide evidence that adenylosuccinate synthetase of brain and testes tissues does not respond to thyroid hormones.

## Materials and Methods

IMP, GTP, $T_4$, and $T_3$ were purchased from Sigma Chemical Company. Universally labelled L-aspartic-$^{14}$C acid (164 mc/mmole) was purchased from New England Nuclear Corporation from Schwarz Biochemical Company. Thyroxine was recrystallized from sodium carbonate and ethanol by a method described by Harington (9). L-$T_3$ was recrystallized in boiling 2N HCL as described by Pitt-Rivers et. al. (13). All stock solutions of thyroxine and L-$T_3$ were prepared in the same manner. They were dissolved in 0.05 ml of 2N NaOH followed by a few drops of water. When they were completely dissolved, they were transferred quantitatively to appropriate volumetric flasks and made up to volume with 0.02 M tris-phosphate buffer, pH 7.6. Further dilutions were then prepared from these stock solutions with buffer.

Tissues for these studies were obtained from growth-arrested, sulfaguanidine-fed male, Sprague-Dawley rats (68). Brain and testes were homogenized with 2.5 volumes of cold, tris-phosphate (0.02M) buffer, pH 7.6, for 30 seconds with a Sorvall homogenizer run at 1/2 maximal speed. The homogenates were centrifuged at

100,000 x g for one hour in a Spinco model L centrifuge. Aliquots

of the supernatant fractions were transferred to incubation tubes.

Radioactivity was measured in a Packard Tri-Carb Liquid

scintillation counter.

Since fumaric acid is also produced when IMP is converted to

AMP, the reaction was conveniently followed by extracting fumaric

acid-$^{14}$C with ether when aspartic acid -$^{14}$C was used as a precursor.

Results

Table 4 shows that thyroid hormones did not inhibit IMP dehydrogenase. Tables 5 and 6 illustrate that thyroid hormones did not stimulate AMP synthesis in brain and testes.

Discussion

These experiments were run to accumulate additional evidence
that the site of action of thyroid hormones is the metabolism of IMP.
The effect of thyroid hormones on adenylosuccinate and IMP dehydrogenase is well correlated with the in vivo effects of the hormones and
their analogues.  Since it had been reported that brain and testes are
not effected by thyroid hormones when administered in vivo, even
in large doses, these tissues provide an additional point of correlation
to test any hypothesis as the site of action of thyroid hormones.  The
effect of thyroid hormones on adenylosuccinate synthetase of brain
and testes had not been tested previously, and these results show
that this enzyme is present in low concentration in these tissues and
it does not respond to either $L-T_3$ or $L-T_4$ as did the liver enzyme.

V.  The effect of thyroid hormones on a microorganism, American

cockroaches and peanuts.

## Introduction

It is an attractive thought to consider the site of action of thyroid hormones is a control of purine synthesis. The response of adenylosuccinate synthetase and IMP dehydrogenase to thyroid hormones is highly correlated with the in vivo effect of the hormones and these reactions would link thyroid hormones to energy production of the cell, allosteric control of certain key enzymes, RNA synthesis and indirectly, with protein synthesis. However, it is difficult to visualize the significance of an inhibition of GMP synthesis. This problem may be formulated more directly: How does an inhibition of GMP synthesis result in an increased basal metabolic rate and a stimulation of growth? Stimulation of basal metabolic rate is a characteristic response to thyroid hormones.

When considered from this point of view, it became apparent that an in vitro system would be necessary for studying the effect of thyroid hormones on purine synthesis and on RNA and protein synthesis. In general, in vitro systems obtained from animal tissue have a relatively short life span. For example, the cytoplasmic protein synthesizing system of rat liver, is capable of incorporating amino acids for approximately 20 minutes. The studies of Tata and Widnell (49) indicate that protein synthesis in rat liver is not stimulated before 30 hours after the administration of thyroid hormones. Thus, the use of animal tissues for studying the effect of thyroid hormones did not offer much promise. It was considered possible that adenylosuccinate synthetase and IMP dehydrogenase of other species may respond to thyroid hormones in a manner similar to that observed in animal tissues. The thyroid gland appeared rather late in the evolution of higher forms of life and it seemed reasonable to expect that the metabolic system of certain lower forms of life would respond to thyroid hormones. If so, lower forms of life may be more useful as models for studying the mechanism of action of thyroid hormones. For example, a single cell grown in the presence of thyroid hormones would produce a colony of cells that would be markedly different from normal cells. In animal tissues, any modification produced by thyroid hormones is diluted by tissue which is already present. In addition, a study of the response of other species other than animal to thyroid hormones is of value in the field of comparative biochemistry.

This section is of an exploratory nature in which the effect of thyroid hormones on yeast, A. aerogenes, Cellvibrio gilvus, American cockroaches and peanuts was investigated.

The effect of thyroid hormones on <u>Saccharomyces cerevisiae</u>,
<u>Cellvibrio gilvus</u> and <u>A. aerogenes</u>.

Experimental

## Culture of microorganisms:

Saccharomyces cerevisiae were grown with aeration on a liquid medium containing (in mg/l): DL-aspartic acid, 400; -alanine, 2; $KH_2PO_4$, 4000; $(NH_4)_2SO_4$, 6000; $MgSO_4 \cdot 7H_2O$, 500; $CaCl_2 \cdot 2H_2O$, 500; KI, 0.2; i-inositol, 10; thiamine-HCl, 0.04; p-amino-benzoic acid, 0.2; nicotinic acid, 0.2; pyridoxal phosphate, 0.04; and sucrose, 40,000. The cells were transferred from agar slants to a tube containing 20 ml of the same medium. These were incubated at $30^\circ$ for 24 hours. The 24 hour culture was used for the growth study and kinetic studies.

## Preparation of sonicate for kinetic studies.

A twenty-four hour culture of yeast was transferred into 3 liters of medium and incubated for 48 hours at $30^\circ$. The yeast suspension were washed once by centrifugation at $0^\circ$ for 20 minutes at 400 x g in 0.05M tris-phosphate buffer at pH 8.3. The washed culture was resuspended in the same buffer and stirred for 10 minutes with a magnetic stirrer to break up the clumps. The cells were resuspended in tris-phosphate buffer and extracts were prepared by sonication (MSE ultrasonic disintegrators, Model DF 101, serial

H-369, V. Raytheon Manufacturing Co.) The duration of sonication

was 15 minutes for each 20 ml of yeast at 1.1 ampers out put current,

at a frequency of 10 KC/sec. Ninety-five per cent of the cells were

broken which was established microscopically. The sonicate was

centrifuged at 100,000 x g for 1 hour. The supernatant was used as

the source of enzymes.

The bacterial cells of Cellvibrio gilvus strain 11 were grown

in a medium containing (in g/l): yeast extract (Difco), 1: casein-

hydrolysate, 0.5; KCl, 0.25; $(NH_4)_2SO_4$ , 0.25; $K_2HPO_4$, 0.5;

cellulose, 1.

A. aerogenes was grown in a medium containing; $K_2HPO_4$,

1.1%; $KH_2PO_4$, 85%; Difco yeast extract, 0.6%, and glucose 1%.

Cultures were grown with vigorous aeration. Three day cultures

of Cellvibrio gilvus were ground for 5 minutes with an amount of

alumina equal to twice the weight of the cells. Then the mixture was

chilled in a mortar and ground with a pestle. The chilled mixture was

ground vigorously for 3-5 minutes. During the grinding the mixture

loses its original dry appearance and becomes pasty. After grinding

is completed, 10 ml of buffer (tris-HCl 0.02M 0.009 M Mg acetate

0.07 M KCl, pH 7.8) was added for each 3 gram of wet cells. The pre-

paration was centrifuged for 10 minutes at 400 x g to remove alumina and

cells and cell debris was then spun at 100,000 x g   for 60 minutes.
The supernatant was adjusted to pH 8.3.

Enzymes.   IMP dehydrogenase for yeast and Cellvibrio
gilvus was purified by the method described for rat liver.

AMP synthesis was studied in the crude supernatant fraction
of the yeast sonicate.

Assays.   IMP dehydrogenase was assayed by measuring the
reduction of NAD at 340 mu as was described in the first section.

The fumarate assay was used to measure the synthesis of
AMP, as was described in the second section.

Growth.   Cells of yeast and A. aerogenes were grown in the
same medium described previously.   The hormone supplements were
dissolved in methanol and $H_2O$ (1:1) and 0.2 ml was added to 20 ml of
culture media after the media had been sterilized.   The tubes were
capped with aluminum caps and autoclaved for 10 minutes and then in-
oculated after cooling by transferring 0.2 ml of the 24 hours culture,
and incubated at different time intervals.   Growth was measured
turbidometerically using a Spectronic 20 at 490 mu.

## Results

Tables 7 and 8 show that IMP dehydrogenase of yeast and Cellvibrio gilvus was purified to approximately the same extent as that obtained from rat liver.

The effect of thyroid hormones: Fig. 15 illustrates that L-$T_3$ inhibits IMP dehydrogenase from yeast maximally at $10^{-5}$M and to lesser extent at $10^{-7}$M, but $10^{-9}$M L-$T_3$ stimulated the reaction slightly. With L-$T_4$ the pattern was somewhat different. The inhibition was maximal at $10^{-5}$M and to a lesser extent at $10^{-7}$M and $10^{-9}$M. This is different from the response of liver enzyme.

Table 9 shows that thyroid hormones had no stimulatory effect on AMP synthesis in yeast extracts.

Table 11 shows that the growth of yeast incubated for 15 hours was stimulated with $10^{-5}$M L-$T_4$. Lower concentrations have no effect or inhibit the growth. A greater stimulatory effect was observed when both L-$T_3$ and L-$T_4$ were incubated for 30 hours.

If microorganisms respond to thyroid hormones, and the site of their action is on IMP-dehydrogenase and adenylosuccinate synthetase, it seemed possible that the effect of thyroid hormones would be simulated by growing the organisms with adenine and guanine in various ratios. To test the effect of purine bases on the growth of the yeast, yeast cells were grown in the presence of adenine and quanine and Table 12 shows that the growth of the yeast was stimulated maximally with a ratio of $\frac{9 \text{ Guanine}}{1 \text{ Adenine}}$ and inhibited maximally when the ratio was $\frac{1 \text{ Guanine}}{10 \text{ Adenine}}$ .

Fig. 16 shows that IMP dehydrogenase of Cellvibrio gilvus was inhibited by $10^{-5}$M L-T$_3$. Lower concentrations and L-T$_4$ had no effect on this enzyme.

Table 10 shows that thyroid hormones control the growth of A. aerogenes. After 15 hours at $10^{-9}$M L-T$_4$ stimulation of growth was maximal and to lesser extent at $10^{-7}$M L-T$_4$. $10^{-5}$M L-T$_4$ had no effect. With L-T$_3$ the effect was similar. $10^{-9}$M L-T$_3$ stimulated the growth more than $10^{-7}$M L-T$_3$. At $10^{-5}$M L-T$_3$ the inhibition is quite clear.

The effect of thyroid hormones on
the American cockroach

Introduction

The American cockroach (Periplaneta americana) was

available at this institution as an experimental animal.

The results of the experiments on certain microorganisms

indicated that it would be worthwhile to test the effect of thyroid

hormones on this insect.

## Experimental

Enzymes. The enzymes used for AMP synthesis were obtained from soluble fractions of the thorax plus abdomen of male American cockroaches which had been adults for at least 7 days. The alimentary canals were carefully removed from both organs to avoid contamination from this source. The wings were removed and immediately after dissection, the isolated thoraces and abdomens were combined and were placed in a beaker containing ice-cold 0.05 M tris-phosphate buffer, weighed and hormogenized in 2.5 volumes (w/v) of cold 0.003 M EDTA. The supernatant fraction was separated from other cell fractions by centrifugation at 100,000 x g for 1 hour in a Spinco refrigerated ultra centrifuge. The resultant supernatant served as the crude enzyme preparation.

IMP dehydrogenase was obtained from the abdomens and was separated from the thoraces, the isolated abdomen were placed in a beaker containing ice-cold 0.05 M tris-phosphate buffer, weighed and homogenized in 2.5 volumes (w/v) of cold 0.003 M EDTA. The enzyme used in these experiments were obtained from soluble fractions of the abdomen of male cockroaches. The supernatant of the homogenate was strained through a cheese cloth and centrifuged out at 100,000 x g for 1 hour in a Spinco refrigerated centrifuge. The resultant supernatant was the starting material for the purification procedure which was prepared by the procedure used for the isolation of the enzyme from rat liver.

Assays. IMP dehydrogenase was assayed by measuring the reduction of NAD at 340 mu as was described in the first section.

The synthesis of AMP was measured by the fumarate assay as was described in the second section.

Growth. Thirty five newly hatched, male American cock-roaches were placed together in a large beaker. During the entire feeding period the food in the food cups was changed every 3 days and roaches were weighed. Distilled water was available at all times. The temperature was approximately $25^o$ during the entire experiment. The diet was composed of the following ( in grams ) ground wheat, 55; crude casein, 8.5; alfalfa leaf meal, 2.0; peanut oil meal, 13.0; brewers yeast, 0.5; refined hydrogenated cotton seed oil, 10:0; sucrose, 8.75; sodium chloride, 0.75; calcium carbonate, 1.5; and crystalline vitamins (in mg); menadione, 0.5; biotin, 0.1; vitamin $B_{12}$, 0.004. This diet contained 19.3% of protein (Kjeldahl N x 6.25) and various levels of thyroid hormones/100 gm of diet. The diet was ground to a fine powder. Cockroaches were weighed at $0^0$ because the use of $CO_2$ caused a high death rate.

Results

Table 13 shows that IMP dehydrogenase of American cock-roaches was purified to approximately the same extent as that obtained from rat liver. Initially the thorax and abdomen were used as a source of enzyme, but subsequent experiments established that the enzyme was located entirely in the abdomen.

The effect of thyroid hormones: Fig. 19 illustrates that $L-T_3$ at $10^{-9}M$, $L-T_4$ at $10^{-7}$ and $L-T_4$ propionate at $10^{-5}M$ inhibited IMP dehydrogenase from abdomen.

Table 14 shows that $10^{-5}M$ and $10^{-7}M$ $L-T_3$ stimulated AMP synthesis but to lesser extent at $10^{-9}M$. The same pattern was observed with $L-T_4$. At $10^{-5}$ and $10^{-7}M$ the reaction was stimulated but less with $10^{-9}M$.

Fig. 18 shows that the growth of these cockroaches was stimulated maximally with 8 ug or 16 ug of $L-T_4/100$ g diet. Lower concentrations had less stimulatory effect. With $L-T_3$ the pattern was different. The maximum response was obtained with 0.5 ug/100 g diet. Higher concentrations had no effect or inhibited the growth.

The effect of thyroid hormones on peanuts.

## Experimental

Enzymes.  Large seeded Virginia type peanut (Arachis hypogaea L.) seeds were dusted with Spergon, a fungicide, and germinated in the dark at $30^o$ for 5 days.  The cotyledons were excised from etiolated peanut seedlings, washed several times with distilled water, and homogenized in 2.5 volumes (w/v) of 0.05 M tris-phosphate pH 8.3 for 1 minute at top speed with a Servall Omni-Mixer.  The homogenate was passed through 4 layers of cheesecloth and centrifuged at 100,000 x g for 1 hour.

The enzymes used for AMP synthesis were obtained from the soluble fraction of the crude homogenates.

IMP dehydrogenase was purified from the supernatant of the crude homogenate, by the method described for rat liver.

Assays.-The fumarate assay procedure was used to measure AMP synthesis and IMP dehydrogenase was assayed by following the reduction of NAD at 340 mu as was described in the first section.

Growth Studies.  Samples of 20 seeds identical in size and weight were soaked for 7 hours in 100 ml of water or water containing thyroid hormones. They were then transferred to petri plates and allowed to germinate at room temperature in the dark. After 5, 10, or 15 days, the length of the stem was measured as an index of the growth.

RNA, protein, lipid isolation. Samples of 10 seeds, identical in weight and size, were preincubated in 50 ml of water or water containing $10^{-5}$M L-$T_3$ for 7 hours. They were then transferred to petri plates and allowed to germinate in the presence of glycine-$^{14}$C, (u. l.), 5 uc; $NaH^{14}CO_3$, 15 uc; L-aspartic-$^{14}$C, (u. l), 15 uc or these precursors plus $10^{-5}$M L-$T_3$ for 48 hours. The cotyledons were excised from etiolated peanut seedlings, washed several times with distilled water, and 1 g of tissue was homogenized in 10 ml of 0.05M tris-phosphate pH 8.3 for 1 minute at top speed using a Servall Omni-Mixer. This was centrifuged in the cold at 500 x g for 10 minutes. The residue of cellular debris was discarded. The crude supernatant was adjusted to 0.2 M $HClO_4$, and the precipitate was washed twice with 10 ml cold 0.2 M $HClO_4$. The combined extracts constitute the acid-soluble phosphorus fraction.

Removal of Lipids. The tissue residue was extracted thrice with 10 ml of ethanol:ether:chloroform (2:2:1), at room temperature.

Extraction of RNA. To the tissue residue 10 ml of 0.3 N potassium hydroxide were added and mixed. After incubation for 20 hours at $37^\circ$C in a water bath, the digest was cooled in ice, and the protein and DNA were precipitated by adding 1.2 ml of 6 N cold $HClO_4$. The quantity of RNA in an aliquot of this solution was determined spectrophotometrically. Another aliquot was neutralized with 0.3 N KOH and counted in a Nuclear Chicago liquid scintillation counter with a counting efficiency of 60% for $^{14}C$.

An alkaline hydrolysate was used as a source for mononucleotides and was subjected to ascending one-dimensional paper chromotography for 20 hours, at room temperature with system No. I, isobutyric acid/conc. $NH_4OH$/water, (66:1:33) pH 3.7. Authentic samples were developed on a separate chromatogram. The Rf's of AMP and GMP were 0.44 and 0.165 respectively. Those spots having Rf's of 0.44 and 0.165 were eluted with 1 M phosphate buffer, pH 7.0 and the eluates were centrifuged. The absorption spectrum of the eluates was measured and measured again after the solutions were made acid by the addition of HCl. These measurements were made against comparable extracts of a blank paper chromatogram developed with the same solvent system.

Estimation of protein. The protein was washed twice with hot ($85-90^\circ$) 10% TCA, twice with hot ($80^\circ$) 95% ethanol and twice with warm ($40-45^\circ$) acetone ether (1:1). The extracted protein precipitate was dried for 30 minutes, at $100^\circ$, and then after cooling to room temperature was weighed. A 1-3 mg portion of each dried sample was weighed with a Cahn electrobalance, quantitatively transferred to a scintillation counting vial and dissolved in 1.0 ml of M hydroxide of hyamine in methanol by recapping the vials and heating at 60° for approximately one hour. To each vial was added 15 ml of scintillator fluid containing 0.4% PPO and 0.01% POPOP in toluene. Counting was then carried out in a Packard Tri-Carb scintillation spectrometer.

Amino acid assays were determined by the method, Moore and Stein (116), by Spackman, Moore and Stein (117). One hundred mg of protein was hydrolyzed in 10 ml of 6 N HCl for 24 hours. The hydrolysis was carried out in a sealed tube and kept at a temperature of 110°. The hydrolysate was filtered and dried by a rotory evaporator at a water bath temperature of 50°. The dry sample was put in a vaccum desiccator with some NaOH pellets to remove HCl and then dissolved in 40 ml of 0.2 Na citrate buffer, pH 2.2, to give a final concentration of 1.25 mg/ml. One ml of this solution was applied to a column of 8% cross lined, sulfonated styrene copolymer ion exchange resin contained in the model 120 B amino acid analyzer. The basic amino acids and ammonia were separated on a column (15 cm) operated at 50° and with the pH 5.28 of 0.3 N Na citrate buffer.

The acidic and neutral amino acids, shown in the long second column, were separated on a column (150 cm) which was also operated at 50°. The elution of the column was started with pH 3.28, 0.2 N Na citrate buffer and then changed to the pH 4.25 0.2N Na citrate according to Spackman et. al. (117).

## Results

Table 15 shows that IMP dehydrogenase of peanuts was purified to approximately the same extent as that obtained from rat liver.

The effect of thyroid hormones: Fig. 20 illustrates that L-T$_3$ at $10^{-9}$M, L-T$_4$ at $10^{-7}$M and L-T$_4$ propionate at $10^{-5}$M inhibited IMP dehydrogenase of peanuts.

Table 16 shows that $10^{-5}$ and $10^{-7}$M L-T$_3$ stimulated AMP synthesis but at $10^{-9}$M there was only a slight stimulation. The same pattern was observed with L-T$_4$, at $10^{-5}$M and $10^{-7}$M, D-T$_4$ at $10^{-5}$M had no stimulatory effect.

Fig. 21 shows that the growth of peanuts was stimulated at $10^{-5}$M L-T$_3$. Lower concentrations had no effect or inhibited the growth. L-T$_4$ and D-T$_4$ inhibited the growth of peanuts.

Table 17 shows that L-T$_3$ stimulated the specific activity of RNA and Table 18 implies that thyroid hormones promote the synthesis of an RNA rich in adenine.

Table 20 shows that the protein synthesis of peanuts was stimulated by L-T$_3$. Table 21 shows that the concentration of some amino acids was enhanced by $L-T_3$, but because of the high salt concentration of the buffer used to elute the amino acids and the presence of ninhydrin in the fractions collected by the Beckman amino acid analyzer, the radioactivity of the various amino acids could not be determined with accuracy. The values shown in Table 21 are therefore considered only as approximate.

The concentration of the protein was high in $L-T_3$ treated sample (Table 21), and this was confirmed by the amino acid analysis (Table 22).

## Discussion

Endocrinologists have been intrigued by the possibility of demonstrating hormonal effects on "primitive," single-celled organisms. In the thyroid field, several early reports concerning enhancement of growth of protozoan cultures by desiccated thyroid substances can be discounted on the basis of the impure material. In general, pure thyroxine had no stimulatory effect and often inhibited growth, as was reported for paramecium by Torrey et al. (86) and for tetrahymena by Wingo and Cameron (87). Thyroxine did accelerate the pulsation of paramecium contractile vacuoles and Leichsenring (88) found the metabolic rate of paramecia increased by desiccated thyroid.

In 1955 Wainfan and Marx (89) reported enhanced oxygen consumption of resting cell suspensions of Aerobacter aerogenes when preincubated with $L-T_3$ or $L-T_4$ or $L-T_4$ propionic acid. Gutenstein and Marx (90) working first with a pure culture of Saccharomyces cerevisiae, then with Fleischmann's Active dry yeast, obtained a response to $T_4$ with great sensitivity.

In section one and two it was established that the response of adenylosuccinate synthetase and IMP dehydrogenase to thyroid hormones in animals is highly correlated with the in vivo effect of these hormones, and these results form the basis of a hypothesis in which thyroid hormones control the energy level of the cell and the synthesis of nucleic acids. A model system to study this hypothesis was needed and so various organisms were tested to obtain an in vitro system in which the various interrelated systems of cell metabolism such as nucleic acid synthesis and protein synthesis could be studied after exposure to thyroid hormones.

Yeast for example was grown in various concentrations of — both $L-T_4$ and $L-T_3$. The growth of the yeast was stimulated at $10^{-5}M$ $L-T_4$ and to lesser extent by $10^{-7}M$ and $10^{-9}M$ $L-T_4$. Theoretically, then, we could produce a culture grown in the presence of thyroid hormones that is different than control cultures in its composition of nucleic acids and enzyme activity. Thyroid hormones inhibited IMP dehydrogenase but these hormones had no effect on AMP synthesis.

The use of yeast may not be a good choice because $L-T_3$ is less effective than $L-T_4$ on growth and IMP dehydrogenase. Adenine inhibited growth and AMP synthesis was not affected by thyroid hormones. But in spite of these reasons one phase of this hypothesis (control of nucleotide synthesis by thyroid hormones) was established, that is growth was stimulated by guanine. It would be very interesting

to study the effect of thyroid hormones on other strains of yeast. If

our hypothesis is true, we would expect thyroid hormones to stimulate

the growth of those yeast with a high adenine content in their nucleic

acids.

Saccharomyces cerevisiae strain 285-A was shown by Abrams

(115) to require either adenine or hypoxanthine for growth and to

develop a pink color on exhaustion of these bases in the medium. The

purine requirement could not be fulfilled by Guanine or xanthine. Such

an organism might be a convenient tool for studying the effect of these

hormones on AMP synthesis.

Although Cellvibrio gilvus and A. aerogenes have responded to

thyroid hormones, more work is needed on various enzymes and on

growth to evaluate its significance.

A number of reports have appeared, describing the occurrence

of thyroid hormone formation in certain insects, annelids and molluscs

(91). Wheeler has noted the accumulation of radioiodine in scleroprotein

form in the hypodermis of larval drosophila (92). Other studies have

demonstrated the formation of thyroid hormones by combining the

sensitive techniques of $I^{131}$ - labelling with paper chromotographic

analysis in cockroaches (91). On the basis of these observations, it has

been suggested that the synthesis of thyroid hormones is widespread in the animal kingdom, that the formation of the thyroid hormones preceded that of the thyroid gland, in phylogeny, and that the distinguishing feature of the thyroid gland is its ability to concentrate iodide. The question which has been asked--Is there any evidence that these hormones have functional significance in cockroaches? Further investigation is necessary. The results have indicated that these hormones inhibited IMP dehydrogenase, stimulated AMP synthesis, and promoted growth. The use of cockroaches may be a good choice because $L-T_3$ was more effective than $L-T_4$.

Thus it may be possible to use cockroaches as a model for studying the effect of thyroid hormones on metabolism.

The effect of thyroid hormones on IMP dehydrogenase, AMP synthesis and growth of peanuts is similar to the effect of thyroid hormones on rat liver. $L-T_3$ was more effective than $L-T_4$ and they were both effective at low concentrations. These effects constitute the basic requirement for use of peanuts as a model to study the mechanism of action of thyroid hormones. Iodinated compounds have been found in plants. Monoiodotyrosine and diiodotyrosine have been found in the marine algae, Laminaria flexicaulis (93) and Nercocytis luetkenana (94).

Other reports have shown that $L-T_4$ at $10^{-5}M$ caused a three to five-fold increase in benzoyl aspartate production of segments of pea epicotyls excised from the apex of the third internode (75).

Peanut cotyledons are the only source which synthesize RNA during seed germination and subsquent growth of the plant (95)(96). The high endogenous ribonuclease activity of the aged cotyledons made it necessary to study the effect of thyroid hormones during the early stages of growth. In the studies reported here, RNA, proteins and lipids were isolated after two days germination in presence and absence of $10^{-5}$M L-$T_3$. When peanuts were grown in the presence of thyroid hormones, the synthesis of RNA proteins and lipid were stimulated. The specific activity of the AMP of RNA was greater than that of the control when peanuts were incubated with L-$T_3$.

An attempt was made to determine the composition of the protein synthesized in peanuts that had been treated with L-$T_3$. The results shows that the concentration of glutamic acid and lysine were affected to a greater extent than other amino acids. More works remain to be done to evaluate the significance of these results.

It is planned to consider further the use of peanuts as a model system.

VI. Discussion

This investigation provides evidence that the thyroid
hormones inhibit GMP synthesis, while previous work has shown
that these hormones stimulate AMP synthesis (52). Two enzymes
which have been partially purified from rat liver have been shown to
be directly affected by thyroid hormones. These are adenylosuccinate
synthetase which catalyzes the conversion of IMP to adenylosuccinate
(65) and IMP dehydrogenase which catalyzes the conversion of IMP to
XMP. Therefore thyroid hormones control the cellular AMP/GMP
ratio by stimulating AMP synthesis concommitant with an inhibition of
GMP synthesis. Since IMP is the common precursor for both AMP
and GMP, these results become important because they indicate that
this branched pathway is subject to the control of thyroid hormones,
and lead us to suggest that these two enzymes are the site of action
of thyroid hormones. Experimental and indirect evidence will be
presented to support this hypothesis.

The idea that hormones control specific enzyme functions in
the cell has been widely accepted. At present no hypothesis has been
put forward to explain the mode of action of the thyroid hormones
which is entirely acceptable. This new hypothesis is acceptable

because it satisfies certain requirements. $L-T_4$, $L-T_3$ acetic acid, $L-T_3$ propionic acid, $L-T_4$ acetic acid all inhibited the enzyme reaction. These compounds are physiologically active. D-thyroxine, $T_2$-propionic acid, $T_2$-tyrosine and $T_2$-thyronine, which are physiologically inactive analogues of thyroid hormones, had no inhibitory effect on IMP dehydrogenase. The same correlation was observed with adenylosuccinate synthetase (65). Those compounds which are physiologically active were capable of stimulating this enzyme and those which are physiologically inactive had little or no effect. Thus there is a correlation between chemical structure and action on enzymes on the one hand and on the whole animal on the other. This correlation is absent in studies on other enzymes. D- and L-T$_4$ which have very different biological activities, uncouple oxidative phosphorylation to about the same extent in vitro (97). The "anti thyroxine" drug n-butyl, 4-hydroxy-3, 5-diiodbenzoate is as potent an uncoupler as thyroxine itself (98). Klemperer (99) has reported that $L-T_4$, $D-T_4$, $T_2$ thyronine and L-thyronine uncouple oxidative phosphorylation to the same degree. The last three compounds have no activity in vivo. Further examples of lack of correlation of in vitro and in vivo effects are apparent in studies with ATPase (25). The physiologically inert DL-"ortho"-T$_4$ and $T_2$ propionic acid were as active in vitro as $L-T_4$ and $L-T_4$, in stimulating succinooxidase or inhibiting malate oxidation (100). Thus, the correlation between the in vivo effects of certain compounds and their effect on IMP-dehydrogenase supports the hypothesis that this enzyme is the site of action of thyroid hormones.

The effect of thyroid hormones on AMP and GMP synthesis represents a physiological rather than a pharmacological action. In order to evaluate the significance of the effect of a thyroid hormone on an enzyme, the concentration of hormone used for eliciting a response in vitro must not be high when compared to the physiological level of the hormone in the tissues. In the experiment, on AMP and GMP synthesis so far discussed, the responses have been obtained in the presence of low concentrations of thyroxine or related substances. The stimulation of adenylosuccinate synthetase is maximal with $10^{-9}$M L-$T_3$ or $10^{-5}$M L-$T_4$. IMP dehydrogenase was inhibited maximally with $10^{-9}$M L-$T_3$ and $10^{-7}$M L-$T_4$. But in the experiments of other investigators, responses have been obtained only in the presence of very high concentrations of thyroxine or related substances or after an animal has been brought to an extreme state of hyperthyroidism. For example, animals have been made thyrotoxic by feeding them a diet incorporating 1-3% of desiccated thyroid (25) or by injection of large doses of thyroxine (101). In some experiments, as much as 28 mg of L-thyroxine has been injected in a rat over a period of 4 days(102).

Such a dose is highly toxic; the animal loses 10% or more of its body weight by the 5th day of treatment.

How a stimulation of AMP synthesis concommitant with an inhibition of GMP synthesis controls metabolism, remains to be determined. Necheles (50) found that thyroid hormones stimulate purine synthesis at $10^{-7}$M and he suggested that the anabolic effect of these hormones on bone marrow may arise in part from the stimulation of purine synthesis. Other evidence has accumulated to show that thyroid hormones act as regulators of nucleic acid synthesis. Finamore and Frieden (103) and Tata (104) found that administration of thyroid hormones to tadpoles stimulated the synthesis of RNA, and Widnell and Tata (49) reported that the administration of $L-T_3$ to thyroidectomized rats stimulated the incorporation of orotic acid-$^{14}$C into nuclear RNA within 3 hours. However, attempts to demonstrate a direct effect of thyroid hormones or nuclear RNA synthesis have not been successful. It is possible that the changes induced in the nucleus were the result of thyroid hormone action outside of the nucleus--possibly as a result of the effect of the hormones on AMP and GMP synthesis. The possibility that the ATP/GTP ratio is a mechanism for directing the synthesis of a specific RNA molecules is supported by Eston, Cory and Frieden (105) who noted a 2-3 fold increase in AMP/GMP labeling pattern of liver RNA after tadpoles had been exposed to $L-T_3$ and injected with $AMP-^{14}C$. They

concluded that a different RNA had been synthesized.

By controlling nucleotide synthesis, the thyroid hormones

may alter the balance of free nucleotides avialable for RNA synthesis.

Such an alternation may influence the synthesis of particular RNA

molecules and specific enzyme proteins, etc. Some support for

this was obtained in the studies with peanuts. RNA synthesis was

enhanced in peanuts treated with $L-T_3$, and the specific activity of

the AMP of RNA was greater than that of the control when peanuts

were incubated with $L-T_3$. To test this hypothesis further, the

nucleotide patterns of the RNA of the nucleus and mitochondria

should be tested. This would help in localizing the effect of the

hormones. Also, the nucleotide patterns of the RNA of the nucleus

and the mitochondria in animal tissue could be tested. The net

effect of a stimulation of AMP synthesis concommitant with an in-

hibition of GMP synthesis would be the maintenance of a high AMP/

GMP ratio. Through a wide concentration range of hormone the con-

centration of AMP relative to GMP would be expected to be high. For

example, when the concentration of $L-T_4$ rises to $10^{-7}M$, the synthesis

of GMP is inhibited, but there would be little stimulation of AMP

synthesis. Then as the concentration of $L-T_4$ increases to $10^{-6}M$ or

$10^{-5}M$, AMP synthesis would be stimulated but GMP synthesis would not be inhibited, and the result would be to increase the concentration of both AMP and GMP with a high AMP/GMP ratio. How the AMP/GMP ratio regulates RNA synthesis is not clear at the present time.

An in vitro system has been devised to test this hypothesis (106). Preliminary experiments have shown that the additions of $L-T_3$ ($10^{-9}M$) to whole rat liver homogenates containing IMP and cofactors necessary for nucleotide synthesis, stimulated incorporation of $-^{14}C$ labelled orotic acid into nuclear RNA. Also it was demonstrated that if nuclei are incubated with $UTP-^{3}H$, CTP and, ATP and GTP in various ratios, a 10/1 ratio of ATP/GTP effected a greater incorporation of $UTP-^{3}H$ into nuclear RNA, than did a 1/1 ratio of ATP/GTP. It seems from this, that the ATP/GTP ratios direct the synthesis of specific RNA molecules. From this it seems reasonable to postulate that a high AMP/GMP ratio promotes the synthesis of RNA rich in adenine. Adenine rich nucleic acids have been isolated from different tissues. Hadjwassilious and Brawerman (107) isolated from rat liver a nucleic acid which was low in guanine and cytosine but high in adenine. The synthesis of such RNA molecules would be seriously affected if the supply of AMP were limited as would occur in hypothyrodism. It may be worthwhile to predict that such a molecule would be absent, or present in low concentrations, in thyroidectomized rats and this RNA would appear rapidly after the administration of thyroid hormones. Salzman, Shatkin, and Sebring

have isolated a mRNA from Hela cells which was high in AMP

relative to GMP (108). The base composition of rRNA from five

mammalian tissue culture strains (109) was determined. Interestingly,

in the five tissues examined, the 28S RNA was characterized by a

relatively high guanine and cytosine and low adenine and uracil. On

the other hand, the low S rRNA fraction had higher adenine and

uracil values and a corresponding decrease in guanine and cytosine.

These results should be compared with those obtained by Montagnier

and Bellamy (110)who isolated two molecular species of ribosomal RNA.

The 16S molecules had a lower guanine and cytosine content than did

the 28S molecules. These findings suggest that there are specific types

of RNA with characterestics that would be expected to be influenced by

thyroid hormones. It remains to be determined whether or not the

synthesis of these RNA molecules is controlled by thyroid hormones.

A selective control of m-RNA synthesis could explain the specificity

of hormonal control. It may be significant that in general animal

tissues have higher $\frac{\text{adenine} + \text{thymine}}{\text{guanine} + \text{cytosine}}$ than do microorganisms.

For example, the DNA of calf thymus has a higher content of adenine

than guanine. Most microorganisms contain DNA which is richer in

guanine than adenine. It is possible that the development of a thyroid

gland and thyroid hormones in the evolutionary process, resulted in a shift in the composition of DNA.

Besides being fundamental structural units for RNA synthesis, purine nucleotides are known to function as specific allosteric effectors for specific enzymes (111). The activity of these enzymes would be altered when the levels of free purine nucleotides are altered in the system. This could be tested by determining the free nucleotide pattern in tissues of rats in different thyroidal states. It is expected to see high AMP/GMP and high ATP/GTP ratios in normal and L-$T_3$-treated rats as compared with tissues from thyroidectomized rats. If the balance of free nucleotides is regulated by thyroid hormones as is proposed, then the activities of certain enzymes would be controlled indirectly by these hormones through the control of purine nucleotides.

In the experiments with peanuts it was noted that thyroid hormones stimulated the synthesis of proteins. This would be in agreement with the numerous reports in which thyroid hormones have been shown to stimulate protein synthesis. Of special interest are the reports of Tatibana and Cohen in which it has been demonstrated that thyroid hormones induce the synthesis of carbamyl phosphate synthetase of tadpole liver (112).

A stimulation of protein synthesis by thyroid hormones appears to be one of the later responses in the sequence of events established by Tata. Cytoplasmic protein synthesis and mitochondrial respiration occurred 18 hours after the administration of $L-T_3$ to thyroidectomized rats (11).

At the present time, there is no reason to believe that the stimulation of protein synthesis is not due to the effect of thyroid hormones on RNA metabolism in the nucleus which in turn may be due to the relative concentration of AMP and GMP.

At the present time it may be worthwhile to speculate on the consequences of different RNA molecules synthesized in response to thyroid hormones as was suggested by Eston et al. (105). It is reasonable to speculate that the newly synthesized RNA is rich in adenine as a result of the high adenine/guanine ratio. If the newly synthesized RNA is messenger RNA, then the protein synthesized on this RNA should be rich in those amino acids whose code words include adenine, for example, lysine. The code word for lysine is AAA (113).

An attempt was made to determine the composition of the protein synthesized in peanuts that had been treated with $L-T_3$. Because of the high salt concentration and the presence of ninhydrin in the fractions collected by the Beckman amino acid analyzer, the specific activity of the various amino acids could not be determined with accuracy. The results are shown in Table 21. These results show that the concentrations of glutamic acid and lysine were affected to a greater extent than other amino acids. More work remains to be done to evaluate the significance of these results. It may be possible to use peanuts as a model system for studying the effect of thyroid hormones on protein synthesis.

It is of interest that certain other microorganisms and cockroaches also responded to thyroid hormones. These should also be considered as possible model systems.

## VIII. Summary

Inosine monophosphate (IMP) is a precursor of the two purine nucleotides, adenosine monophosphate (AMP) and guanosine monophosphate (GMP): IMP $\Longrightarrow$ adenylosuccinate $\longrightarrow$ AMP and IMP $\longrightarrow$ xanthine monophosphate (XMP) $\Longrightarrow$ GMP. The reaction IMP $\longrightarrow$ adenylosuccinate is catalyzed by adenylosuccinate synthetase which was purified by $(NH_4)_2 SO_4$ precipitation and by passage through DEAE-Sephadex, and the reaction IMP $\Longrightarrow$ XMP is catalyzed by IMP dehydrogenase which was purified in a manner similar to adenylosuccinate synthetase. These two enzymes which are affected by thyroid hormones have been studied. Adenylosuccinate synthetase of rat liver is stimulated maximally with $10^{-9}$M L-$T_3$ or $10^{-5}$M L-$T_4$, but not by D-$T_4$, and the effect of other analogues paralled their _in vivo_ effects. The enzyme, IMP dehydrogenase, is inhibited by thyroid hormones, but not by D-$T_4$, and also, the effects of other analogues paralleled their _in vivo_ effects. Further correlation to _in vivo_ studies was obtained from brain and testes tissues. AMP and GMP synthesis were not affected by thyroid hormones. The very low effective concentration of the hormones on these enzyn s, the ineffectiveness of physiologically inactive thyronine derivatives, the ineffectiveness of these hormones on these enzymes from brain and testes, and the importance of these enzymes to energy and nucleic acid metabolism fits the concept of a site of action for thyroid hormones better than many previous suggestions.

These results form the basis of a hypothesis in which thyroid hormones control the energy (ATP) level of the cell and control the synthesis of nucleic acids in the nucleus. A model system to study this was needed and so various organisms were tested for their response to thyroid hormones. Yeast, cockroaches, and peanuts were stimulated (growth) by thyroid hormones. The two enzymes were isolated from these organisms and their response to thyroid hormones tested. The two enzymes from peanuts behaved in a manner similar to the rat enzymes. When peanuts were grown in the presence of thyroid hormones, the specific activity of AMP and GMP was such that it supported the theory that AMP should be high and GMP should be low. It is planned to consider further the use of peanuts as a model system and to investigate the effect of thyroid hormones on the synthesis of RNA and protein in the nucleus.

## X.  References

1.  Wharton, T., Adrenographia: sive, glandularum totius corporis descriptio, London. (cited in Harington, C. R., The Thyroid Gland, Its Chemistry and Physiology, Oxford University Press, London (1933).

2.  Harington, C. R., The Thyroid Gland, Its Chemistry and Physiology.  Oxford University Press, London (1913).

3.  Courtois, B., Ann. Chim., 88, 304, 1813. (cited in Pitt-Rivers, R., and Tata, J. A., The Thyroid Hormones, Pergamon Press, London (1959).

4.  FyFe, A., Edin, Phil, J. 1, 254(1819). (cited in Harington, C. R., The Thyroid Gland, Its Chemistry and Physiology, Oxford University Press, London, 1933).

5.  Coindet, J. R., Decouvr. d. Rem. contre le Goitre. Bibl. Universelle de Geneve (1820). (cited in Harington, C. R., The Thyroid Gland, Its Chemistry and Physiology, Oxford University Press, London (1913).

6.  Kocher, T., Arch. Klin. Chir. 29, 254, 1819. (cited in The Thyroid Gland. Butterworths, London, 1964, Vol. I.).

7.  Baumann, E., Ztschr. Phys. Chem., 21, 319(1896). (cited in The Thyroid Gland, Butterworths, London, 1964, Vol. I. ).

8.  Kendall, E. C., J. Amer. Med. Ass. 64, 2042 (1915).

9.  Harington, C. R., Biochem. J., 20, 293 (1926).

10. Gross, J., Pitt-Rivers, R., Biochem. J., 53, 645(1953).

11. Tata, J. R., Ernester, L., Lindberg, O., Biochem. J., 86, 408 (1963).

12. Barker, S. B., Physiol. Rev., 31, 205 (1951).

13. Pitt-Rivers, R. and Tata, J. The Thyroid Hormones, Pergamon Press, London, 1959, p. 15.

14. Barker, S. B., in "The Thyroid Gland." ed. by Pitt-Rivers, R., and Trotter R., Butterworths, London, 1964, p. 199.

15. Flock, E. V., Bollman, J. L. and Berkson, J., Am. J. Physiol. 155, 402 (1948).

16. Steinheimer, R., Endocrinology, 25, 899(1939).

17. Karp, A., and Stetten, D. , J. Biol. Chem., 179, 819 (1949).

18. Fletcher, K., and Myant, N. B., J. Physiology, 143, 353 (1959).

19. Wilkins, L. Rec. Progr. Hormone Res. 2, 391 (1948).

20. Rowlands, I. W., J. Endocrin. 4, 305 (1944).

21. Gudernastsch, J. F., Arch. Entwicklungsmech. Organ., 35, 457 (1912). (cited in Kendall, E. C., Thyroxine, Monograph Series No. 47, 1929, p. 156).

22. Lynn, W., and Wachowski, H., Quart. Rev. Biol. 26, 123(1951).

23. Fraser, R., J. Exptl. Z001., 133, 519(1956).

24. Paasch, G., and Reinwein, H., Biochem. Z., 211, 468(1929). (cited in Kendall, E. C., Thyroxine, Monograph Series No. 47, 1929, p. 108).

25. Lardy, H. A., and Maley, G. F., Rec. Progr. Hormone Res. 10, 129(1954).

26. Maley, G. F., Amer. J. Physiol. 188, 35(1957).

27. Tapley, D. F., J. Biol. Chem., 222, 325(1956).

28. Tapley, D. F., Cooper, C., and Lehninger, A. L.,
    Biochim. Biophys. Acta., 18, 597(1955).

29. Rall, J. E., and Michel, R., J. Biol. Chem., 238, 1848
    (1963).

30. Rall, J. E. and Pearson, O. H., J. Clin. Endocrinol.,
    16, 1299(1956).

31. Lardy, H. A., and Wellman H., J. Biol. Chem.,
    195, 215(1952).

32. Klemperer, H. G., Biochem. J., 60, 128(1955).

33. Bronk, J. R., and Bronk, M. S., J. Biol. Chem.,
    237, 897(1962).

34. DuToit, C. H., A Symposium on Phosphorus Metabolism
    (John Hopkins Press, Baltimore, Md., 1952), Vol. 2, p. 597.

35. Sokoloff, L., and Kaufman, S., Science, 129, 569(1959).

36. Sokoloff, L., and Kaufman, S., J. Biol. Chem.,
    236, 795 (1961).

37. Sokoloff, L., Kaufman, S., Campbell, P. L., Francis, C. M.,
    and Gelboin, H. V., J. Biol. Chem., 237, 1432 (1963).

38. Weiss, W. P., and Sokoloff, L., Science, 140, 1324(1963).

39. Sokoloff, L., Francis, G. M., and Campbell, P. L.,
    Proc. Nat. Sci., 52, 728 (1964).

40. Stein, O., and Gross, J., Proc. Soc. Exptl. Biol. Med.,
    109, 817(1962).

41. Hanson, R. W., Lindsay, R. H., and Barker, S. B.,
    Biochim. Biophys. Acta, 68, 134(1963).

42. Roodyn, D. B., Freeman, K. B., Tata, J. R., in press. (cited in Thyroid Hormones and Regulation of Protein Synthesis by J. R. Tata).

43. Frieden, E., Am. Zool, 1, 115(1961).

44. Frieden, E., and Mathews, H., Arch. Biochem. Biophys., 73, 107(1958).

45. Herner, A., and Frieden, E., J. Biol. Chem., 235, 2845(1960).

46. Freeman, K., Roodyn, D. B. and Tata, J. R., Biochim. et. Biophys. Acta., 72, 127(1963).

47. Widnell, C. C., and Tata, J. R., Biochim. et. Biophys. Acta., 72, 506(1963).

48. Widnell, C. C., and Tata, J. R., Biochem. J., 92, 313(1964).

49. Widnell, C. C., and Tata, J. R., Biochem. J., 98, 604(1966).

50. Necheles, T. F., Am. J. Physiol. 203, 693(1963).

51. Mah, V., and Ackerman, C. J., Biochem. Biophys. Res. Communications, 17, 326(1964).

52. Mah, V., and Ackerman, C. J., Life Science, 4, 573(1965).

53. Greenberg, R. G., J. Am. Chem. Soc., 74, 6307(1952).

54. Buchanan, J. M., and Schulman, M. P., J. Biol. Chem., 202, 241(1953).

55. Magasanik, B., Moyed, H. S., and Gehring, L. B., J. Biol. Chem., 226, 339(1957).

56. Moyed, H. S., and Magasanik, B., J. Biol. Chem., 226, 351(1957).

57. Abrams, R., and Bently, M., Arch. Biochem. Biophys., 79, 91(1959).

58. Lagerkvist, U., J. Biol. Chem., 233,138(1958).

59. Lagerkvist, U. , J. Biol. Chem. 233,142(1958).

60. Abrams, R., and Bently, M., J. Am. Chem. Soc.,
    77,4179(1955).

61. Gehring, L. B., and Magasanik, B. J., Am. Chem. Soc.,
    77,4685 (1955).

62. Turner, J. F., and King. J. E., Biochemical J.,
    79,147(1962).

63. Carter, C. E., and Cohen, L. H., J. Biol. Chem.,
    222,17(1956).

64. Liberman, I., J. Am. Chem. Soc., 78,251(1956).

65. Mah, V. and Ackerman, C. J., unpublished data.

66. Harington, C. R., Biochem. J., 20,293(1926).

67. Gross, J., and Pitt-Rivers, R., Biochemical J.,
    53,645(1953).

68. Ackerman, C. J., J. Nutrition, 79,140(1963).

69. Hurlbert, R. B., Schmitz, H., Brumm, A. F., and
    Potter, V. R., J. Biol. Chem., 20923(1954).

70. Kornberg, A., and Horecker, B. L., In Snell, E. E. (ed.)
    Biochemical Preparations, Vol. 3, J. Wiley and Sons,
    New York. 1953, p. 23.

71. Warburg, O. and Christian, W., Biochemical, Z.,
    310, 384(1942).

72. Clarke, E. C., and Ball, E. G., Fed. Proc., 14,193(1955).

73. Wolff, E. C., and Ball, E. G., J. Biol. Chem.,
    224,1083 (1957).

74. Hannon, J. P., Fed. Proc., 19, suppl. 5,139(1966).

75. Venis, M. A., Nature, 210, 534(1966).

76. Sugisawa, Endocrinol. Japan, 3, 186(1956). (cited in Pitt-Rivers, R. and Tata, J., The Thyroid Hormones, Pergamon Press, London, 1959, p. 15).

77. Gemmill, G. L., J. Biol. Chem., 192, 749 (1951).

78. Cameron, A. T., and Carmichel, Jr., J. Biol. Chem., 46, 35(1921).

79. Simpson, G. K. and Johnston, A. G., Biochem. J., 41, 181(1947).

80. Crispell, K. R., Williams, G. A., and Parson, W., J. Clin. Endocrinol. Metab., 17, 221(1957).

81. Lawson, K., J. Embryol. Exptl. Morphol., 11, 383(1963).

82. Wellby, M. and M. W. O'Halloran, Brit. Med. J., 2, 668(1966).

83. Money, W. L., Kumanoka, S., Rawson, R. W., and Kroc, R. L., Ann. NY. Acad. Sci., 86, 512(1960).

84. Thibault, O., Arch. Sci. Physiol., 10, 423(1956).

85. Gordon, E. S., and Heming, A. E., Endocrinology, 34, 353(1944).

86. Torrey, H. B., Riddle, M. C., and Brodie, J. L., J. Gen. Physiol., 449(1924).

87. Wingo, W. J., and Cameron, L. E., Texas reports Biol. Med., 10, 1074(1952).

88. Leichsenring, J. M., Am. J. Physiol., 75, 84(1925).

89. Wainfan, E., and Marx, W., J. Biol. Chem., 214, 599(1955).

90. Gutenstein, M., and Marx, W., J. Biol. Chem., 229, 599(1957).

91. Gorbman, A., Clements, M., and Obrien R., J. Exp. Zool. 127, 75(1954).

92. Wheeler, B. M., J. Exp. Zool, 115, 83(1950).

93. Roche, J., and Yagi, Y., Compt. rend. Soc. Biol, 143, 1327(1949).

94. Tong, W., and Chaikoff, I. L., J. Biol. Chem., 215, 473(1955).

95. Cherry, J. H., Plant Physiol., 38, 440(1963).

96. Marcus, A., and Feely, J., Biochim, Biochim. Biophys. Acta 61, 830(1962).

97. Bain, J. A., J. Pharmacol., 110, 2(1954).

98. Hock, J. F., and Lipmann, F., Proc. Natl. Acad. Sci. 40, 909(1954).

99. Klemperer, H. G., Biochem. J., 60, 128(1955).

100. Hamburg, M., and Flexner, L. B., J. Neurochem. 1, 279(1957).

101. Kuby, S. B., Noda, L., and Lardy, H. A., J. Biol. Chem., 210, 65(1954).

102. Dutoit, C. H., Phosphorus Metabolism, Vol. II., p. 597 Ed. W. D. McElroy and B. Glass., John Hopkins Press, Baltimore (1952).

103. Finamore, F. J. and Frieden, E., J. Biol. Chem., 235, 1751(1960).

104. Tata, J. R., Nature (London) 207, 378(1965).

105. Eston, J. E., J. E. Cory and Frieden E., Fed. Proc. 26, 392(1967). Abstract.

106. Lo, R. C. and Ackerman, C. J., unpublished data.

107. Hadjivassiliou, A. and Brawerman, G., Biochim. Biophys. Acta 103, 211(1965).

108. Salzman, N. P., Shatkin, A. J. and Sebring, E. D., J. Mol. Biol., 8, 405(1964).

109. Brown, F., and Martin, S. J., Biochem. J., 79, 20C(1965).

110. Montagnier, J. and Bellamy, J., Biochim. Biophys. Acta 80, 157(1964).

111. Atkinson, D. E., Science, 150, 851(1965).

112. Tatibana, M., and Cohen, P. P., J. Biol. Chem. 239, 2905(1964).

113. Speyer, J. E., Lengyel, Basilio, C., Wahba, Gardner, R. S., and Ochoa, S., Cold Spring Harbor Symp. Quant. Biol., 28, 559(1963).

114. Lee, N. D., Henry, R. J. and Golub, O., J. Clin. Endocr. 24, 486(1964).

115. Abrams, R., Arch. Biochem. Biophys. 37, 270(1952).

116. Moor, S., and Stein, W. H., Method in Enzymology, S. Colowick and N. O. Kaplan (eds.) Academic Press, New York, 1963, Vol. VI, p. 819.

117. Spackman, D. H.; Stein, W. H.; Moore, S. : Anal. Chem., 30, 1190(1958).

XII. Appendices

## TABLE 1

### Purification of IMP dehydrogenase.

| Step Number | Purification Step | Total Activity Units (mu moles NADH/min.) | Total Protein | Specific activity units/mg | Fold Puri- faction |
|---|---|---|---|---|---|
| 1 | acetone powder extract | 0.09 | 2.7 | 0.033 | 1 |
| 2 | ammonium sulfate (30-40%) | 0.3 | 1.5 | 0.2 | 6 |
| 3 | DEAE Sphedex | 0.4 | 0.35 | 1.14 | 34 |

The reaction mixture contained (in umoles): NAD, 14.7; IMP, 19.8; tris-phosphate, pH 8.3, 50; and protein as described in each experiment. The total volume was 1.5 ml. The enzymes were obtained from the livers of normal rats and purified as described in the text. The reaction was followed at 340 mu in spectrophotometer cuvettes for 15 minutes against a blank which contained all ingredients except enzyme.

## TABLE  2

Identification and recovery of xanthine.

| | Maxima | 250/260 | 280/260 | Total xanthine synthesized u moles |
|---|---|---|---|---|
| | | control | | |
| pH 10 | 241, 276 | 1. 26 | 1. 76 | 1. 86 |
| pH 2 | 265 | 0. 67 | 0. 63 | |
| | | control + L-T$_3$, $10^{-9}$M | | |
| pH 10 | 242, 276 | 1. 24 | 1. 75 | 0. 91 |
| pH 2 | 264 | 0. 63 | 0. 62 | |
| | | control + L-T$_4$, $10^{-7}$M | | |
| pH 10 | 242, 274 | 1. 22 | 1. 81 | 0. 60 |
| pH 2 | 266 | 0. 60 | 0. 63 | |
| | | control + xanthine * | | |
| pH 10 | 242, 276 | 1. 24 | 1. 75 | |
| pH 2 | 266 | 0. 61 | 0. 61 | |

* xanthine (0. 1 u mole) was added to an aliquot of the hydrolysate of the control sample just prior to chromotography.

The enzyme preparation and incubation condition were described under Table 1, with 0. 6 mg of protein and with L-T$_3$ or L-T$_4$ as indicated above.  After 15 minutes incubation, the media were hydrolyzed and the hydrolysates developed on paper chromatograms with 90% ethanol: 1. 0 M  NH$_4$-acetate, pH 7. 6 (7:3).  The spots corresponding to xanthine were eluted and the spectra were determined at pH 10 and 2.

## TABLE 3

Summary of the effect of thyroid hormones and certain analogues of L-thyroxine on IMP dehydrogenase of rat liver.

| Compound | mg protein | Concentration | | | | % inhibition at the maxima |
| --- | --- | --- | --- | --- | --- | --- |
| | | 0.0 | $10^{-9}$M | $10^{-7}$M | $10^{-5}$M | |
| | | mu moles | NADH/mg protein/15 min. | | | |
| D-$T_4$ | 0.24 | 3.75 | 3.6 | 3.7 | 5.1 | 4% |
| 3,5-diiodo-L-tyrosine | 0.25 | 4.0 | 4.2 | 4.7 | 3.0 | 25% |
| 3,5-diiodo-L-thyronine | 0.25 | 3.7 | 3.8 | 5.0 | 4.2 | 00% |
| 3,5-diiodothyro-proprionate | 0.60 | 11.2 | 10.5 | 10.7 | 11.7 | 7% |
| 3,5,3',5',-tetraiodo-thyroacetate | 0.23 | 3.6 | 3.4 | 3.1 | 2.6 | 28% |
| 3,5,3',5',-tetraiodo-thyroproprionate | 0.22 | 3.4 | 2.4 | 2.1 | 0.7 | 80% |
| 3,5,3'-triiodothyro-proprionate | 0.6 | 11.1 | 10.7 | 3.2 | 1.6 | 86% |
| L-$T_4$ | 0.22 | 2.8 | 1.3 | 0.8 | 2.75 | 75% |
| L-$T_3$ | 0.30 | 4.0 | 2.7 | 3.6 | 3.9 | 32% |

The incubation media were as described under Table 1, except that the protein concentration for each experiment was as indicated. The enzymes were obtained from normal rats, precipitated with $(NH_4)_2SO_4$ and treated with Sephadex as described in the text.

## TABLE 4

The effect of thyroid hormones on IMP-dehydrogenase of rat brain and testes.

| Exp. | Compound | mg protein | 0.0 | $10^{-9}$M | $10^{-7}$M | $10^{-5}$M |
|------|----------|-----------|-----|-----------|-----------|-----------|
| | | | mu moles | NADH/mg protein /15 min. | | |
| I. Brain | $L\text{-}T_4$ | 0.25 | 3.3 | 4.7 | 5.4 | 5.6 |
| | $L\text{-}T_3$ | 0.25 | 3.3 | 4.7 | 4.7 | 5.1 |
| II. Brain | $L\text{-}T_4$ | 1.2 | 1.3 | 1.4 | 1.4 | 1.5 |
| | $L\text{-}T_3$ | 1.2 | 1.3 | 1.4 | 1.5 | 1.7 |
| III. Testes | $L\text{-}T_4$ | 0.5 | 4.5 | 4.3 | 4.2 | 4.0 |
| | $L\text{-}T_3$ | 0.5 | 4.5 | 4.0 | 4.0 | 4.0 |
| IV. Testes | $L\text{-}T_4$ | 4.5 | 0.56 | 0.54 | 0.54 | 0.50 |
| | $L\text{-}T_3$ | 4.5 | 0.56 | 0.50 | 0.49 | 0.51 |

The incubation media were as described under Table 1, except that the protein concentration for each experiment was as indicated. The enzyme for these experiments was the crude preparation obtained from tissues of growth-arrested, sulfaguanidine-fed rats.

TABLE  5

The effect of thyroid hormones on AMP synthesis in testes.

| Additions | Fumaric acid-$^{14}$C Total cpm/mg protein |
|---|---|
| Complete | 2487 |
| Complete + $10^{-5}$M  L-T$_3$ | 2106 |
| Complete + $10^{-7}$M  L-T$_3$ | 2230 |
| Complete + $10^{-9}$M  L-T$_3$ | 2153 |
| Complete + $10^{-5}$M  L-T$_4$ | 2228 |
| Complete + $10^{-7}$M  L-T$_4$ | 2314 |
| Complete + $10^{-9}$M  L-T$_4$ | 2156 |

Complete system:  0.33 ml of the 100,000  x  g  supernatant of testes; tris-phosphate buffer, pH 7.6, 20 umoles; and in umoles: MgCl$_2$, 2.5; GTP,1; IMP, 5; and L-asparate-u-$^{14}$C, 100,000 cpm in a total volume of 1.0 ml.  Hormones added as noted.  Total protein was 2 mg.  Incubation in air at 37$^{\mathrm{o}}$ for 20 minutes.  All incubations were carried out in duplicate.  After incubation, 0.1 ml of concentrated HCl was added and each tube extracted with ethyl ether for 14 hours in a liquid-liquid extractor.  The ether extract (fumaric acid-$^{14}$C) was counted for radioactivity.

TABLE   6

The effect of thyroid hormones on AMP synthesis in brain.

| Additions | Fumaric acid-$^{14}$C Total cpm/mg protein |
|---|---|
| Complete | 4334 |
| Complete + $10^{-5}$M   L-T$_3$ | 3902 |
| Complete + $10^{-7}$M   L-T$_3$ | 4016 |
| Complete + $10^{-9}$M   L-T$_3$ | 4611 |
| Complete + $10^{-5}$M   L-T$_4$ | 4364 |
| Complete + $10^{-7}$M   L-T$_4$ | 4467 |

The conditions were as described in Table 5. Thyroid hormones were added as indicated. Total protein was 1 mg.

TABLE 7

Purification of IMP dehydrogenase of the yeast.

| Step Number | Purification Step | Total Activity Units (mu moles NADH/min.) | Total Protein | Specific activity units/mg | Fold Puri- fication |
|---|---|---|---|---|---|
| 1 | acetone powder extract | 0.04 | 2.5 | 0.014 | 1 |
| 2 | ammonium sulfate fractionation (30-40%) | 0.09 | 1.25 | 0.072 | 10 |
| 3 | DEAE Sphedex | 0.15 | 0.30 | 0.50 | 35 |

The reaction mixture contained (in umoles): NAD, 14.7; IMP, 19.8; tris-phosphate, pH 8.3, 50; and protein as described in each experiment. The total volume was 1.5 ml. The enzymes were obtained from yeast sonicate and purified as described in the text. The reaction was followed at 340 mu in spectrophotometer cuvettes for 15 minutes against a blank which contained all ingredients except enzyme.

TABLE 8

Purification of IMP dehydrogenase of Cellvibrio gilvus.

| Step Number | Purification Step | Total Activity Units (mu moles NADH/min.) | Total Protein | Specific Activity units/mg | Fold Purification |
|---|---|---|---|---|---|
| 1 | acetone powder extract | 0.08 | 3.5 | 0.022 | 1 |
| 2 | ammonium sulfate fractionation (30-40%) | 0.17 | 1.70 | 0.100 | 4.5 |
| 3 | DEAE Sphedex | 0.28 | 0.32 | 0.84 | 38 |

The reaction mixture contained (in umoles): NAD, 14.7; IMP, 19.8; tris-phosphate, pH 8.3, 50; and protein as described in each experiment. The total volume was 1.5 ml. The enzymes were obtained from Cell vibrio gilvus and purified as described in the text. The reaction was followed at 340 mu in spectrophotometer cuvettes for 15 minutes against a blank which contained all ingredients except enzyme.

TABLE   9

The effect of thyroid hormones in AMP synthesis of the yeast.

| Additions | Fumaric acid-$^{14}$C cpm/mg   protein |
|---|---|
| Complete | 11303 |
| Complete + $10^{-5}$M   L-T$_3$ | 10842 |
| Complete + $10^{-7}$M   L-T$_3$ | 10288 |
| Complete + $10^{-9}$M   L-T$_3$ | 10609 |
| Complete + $10^{-5}$M   L-T$_4$ | 10859 |
| Complete + $10^{-7}$M   L-T$_4$ | 10024 |
| Complete + $10^{-9}$M   L-T$_4$ | 10517 |
| Complete + $10^{-5}$M   L-D$_4$ | 10979 |

Complete system: 0.33 ml of the 100,000  x  g  supernatant of sonicated yeast cells with 1 mg total protein; tris-phosphate buffer, pH 7.6, 20 u moles, and in u moles: $MgCl_2$, 2.5; GTP, 1; IMP, 5; and L-aspartate, 100,000 cpm in a total volume of 1.0 ml.  Hormones added as noted.  Incubation in air at 37° for 20 minutes.  All incubations carried out in duplicate.  After incubation, 0.3 ml of concentrated HCl were added and each tube was extracted with ether for 14 hours in liquid-liquid extractors.  The ether extract (fumaric acid-$^{14}$C) was counted for radioactivity.

TABLE 10

The effect of thyroid hormones on the growth of A. aerogenes.

| Hormone Concentration | L-T$_4$ $\triangle$ A 490 mu | L-T$_3$ $\triangle$ A 490 mu |
|---|---|---|
| 0.00 | 0.350 ± 0.010 | 0.350 ± 0.010 |
| 10$^{-9}$ M | 0.375 ± 0.005 | 0.375 ± 0.005 |
| 10$^{-7}$ M | 0.360 ± 0.005 | 0.360 ± 0.005 |
| 10$^{-5}$ M | 0.325 ± 0.005 | 0.312 ± 0.005 |

Growth of A. aerogenes in the presence of L-T$_4$ and L-T$_3$. Growth was measured at 7.5, 15, and 22.5 hrs. Only the results obtained at 22.5 hrs. are shown.

## TABLE 11

The effect of thyroid hormones on the growth of yeast.

| Hormone concentration | Growth response, 15 hrs. range. | |
|---|---|---|
| | L-T$_4$ $\Delta$ A 490 mu | L-T$_3$ $\Delta$ A 490 mu |
| 0.00 | 0.065 ± 0.010 | 0.065 ± 0.010 |
| 10$^{-10}$M | 0.027 ± 0.006 | 0.037 ± 0.010 |
| 10$^{-9}$ M | 0.045 ± 0.010 | 0.035 ± 0.010 |
| 10$^{-7}$ M | 0.050 ± 0.010 | 0.025 ± 0.010 |
| 10$^{-5}$ M | 0.125 ± 0.010 | 0.010 ± 0.010 |
| | Growth response, 30 hrs. ± range. | |
| 0.00 | 0.100 ± 0.010 | 0.100 ± 0.010 |
| 10$^{-10}$M | 0.087 ± 0.006 | 0.089 ± 0.004 |
| 10$^{-9}$ M | 0.107 ± 0.005 | 0.124 ± 0.004 |
| 10$^{-7}$ M | 0.206 ± 0.006 | 0.183 ± 0.003 |
| 10$^{-5}$ M | 0.355 ± 0.006 | 0.105 ± 0.005 |

Growth of Saccharomyces cerevisiae in the presence of L-T$_4$ and L-T$_3$. Growth was measured at 490 mu after 0, 15, 30 and 45 hours. Only 15 and 30 hour results are shown.

## TABLE 12

The influence of adenine and guanine on the growth of yeast.

| Quanine | Adenine | A:G | Growth response $\Delta$ A 490 mu |
|---|---|---|---|
| 0.00 | 0.00 | 0:0 | .250 $\pm$ 0.010 |
| $10^{-4}$M | $10^{-4}$M | 1:1 | .250 $\pm$ 0.012 |
| 3 x $10^{-4}$M | 0.00 | 0:1 | .300 $\pm$ 0.005 |
| 3 x $10^{-4}$M | $10^{-4}$M | 1:3 | .325 $\pm$ 0.005 |
| 6 x $10^{-4}$M | $10^{-4}$M | 1:6 | .350 $\pm$ 0.00t |
| 9 x $10^{-4}$M | $10^{-4}$M | 1:9 | .350 $\pm$ 0.005 |
| $10^{-4}$M | 3 x $10^{-4}$M | 3:1 | .250 $\pm$ 0.005 |
| 0.00 | $10^{-4}$M | 1:0 | .225 $\pm$ 0.005 |
| $10^{-4}$M | 10 x $10^{-4}$M | 10:1 | .225 $\pm$ 0.005 |

Growth of Saccharomyces cerevisiae in the presence of adenine ranging from $10^{-4}$M to 9 x $10^{-4}$M and guanine from $10^{-4}$M to 10 x $10^{-4}$M. Growth was measured at 490 mu at 25 hours.

## TABLE 13

Purification of IMP dehydrogenase from American cockroaches.

| Step Number | Purification Step | Total Activity units (mu moles NADH/ min.) | Total Protein | Specific Activity units/mg | Fold Puri- fication |
|---|---|---|---|---|---|
| 1 | acetone powder extract | 0.04 | 3.0 | 0.013 | 1 |
| 2 | ammonium sulfate fractionation (30-40%). | 0.10 | 1.5 | 0.066 | 5 |
| 3 | DEAE Sphedex | 0.15 | 0.35 | 0.42 | 32 |

The reaction mixture contained (in umoles): NAD, 14.7; IMP, 19.8; tris-phosphate, pH 8.3, 50; and protein as described in each experiment. The total volume was 1.5 ml. The enzymes were obtained from the abdomen of American cockroaches and purified as described in the text. The reaction was followed at 340 mu in spectrophotometer cuvettes for 15 minutes against a blank which contained all ingredients except enzyme.

## TABLE 14

The effect of thyroid hormones on AMP synthesis in American cockroaches.

| Additions | cpm/mg protein |
|---|---|
| Complete | 2623 |
| Complete + $10^{-5}$M L-T$_3$ | 3820 |
| Complete + $10^{-7}$M L-T$_3$ | 3650 |
| Complete + $10^{-9}$M L-T$_3$ | 3290 |
| Complete + $10^{-5}$M L-T$_4$ | 3670 |
| Complete + $10^{-7}$M L-T$_4$ | 3310 |
| Complete + $10^{-9}$M L-T$_4$ | 3100 |

The conditions were as described in Table 5, except that the enzymes were prepared from the supernatant of the abdomen and thorax crude homogenates. Total protein was 2 mg.

## TABLE 15

Purification of IMP dehydrogenase from peanuts.

| Step Number | Purification Step | Total Activity Units (mu moles NADH/min.) | Total Protein | Specific Activity units/mg | Fold Puri- fication |
|---|---|---|---|---|---|
| 1 | acetone powder extract | 0.08 | 3.5 | 0.022 | 1 |
| 2 | ammonium sulfate fractionation (30-40%) | 0.16 | 1.5 | 0.10 | 4.4 |
| 3 | DEAE Sphedex | 0.26 | 0.38 | 0.60 | 30.9 |

The reaction mixture contained (in umoles): NAD, 14.7; IMP 19.8; tris-phosphate, pH 8.3, 50; and protein as described in each experiment. The total volume was 1.5 ml. The enzymes were obtained from peanuts and purified as described in the text. The reaction was followed at 340 mu in spectrophotometer cuvettes for 15 minutes against blank which contained all ingredients except enzyme.

TABLE 16

The effect of thyroid hormones on AMP synthesis in peanuts.

| Additions | Fumaric acid -$^{14}$C cpm/mg protein |
|---|---|
| Complete | 2128 |
| Complete + $10^{-5}$M  L-T$_3$ | 3595 |
| Complete + $10^{-7}$M  L-T$_3$ | 3385 |
| Complete + $10^{-9}$M  L-T$_3$ | 2400 |
| Complete + $10^{-5}$M  L-T$_4$ | 3200 |
| Complete + $10^{-7}$M  L-T$_4$ | 2786 |
| Complete + $10^{-9}$M  L-T$_4$ | 2095 |
| Complete + $10^{-5}$M  D-T$_4$ | 2113.4 |

The conditions were as described in Table 5, except that the enzymes were prepared from the supernatant of the peanut crude homogenate. Total protein was 2 mg.

TABLE   17

The effect of triiodo-L-thyronine on RNA synthesis in peanuts.

| Addition | $\dfrac{\text{cpm}}{\text{g tissue}}$ | $\dfrac{\text{ug RNA}}{\text{g tissue}}$ | $\dfrac{\text{cpm}}{\text{ug RNA}}$ |
|---|---|---|---|
| | | RNA, 48 hours | |
| None | 20738 | 502.8 | 41.2 |
| L-T$_3$ | 30964 | 490.8 | 63 |
| | | RNA, 96 hours | |
| None | 36738 | 680 | 54 |
| L-T$_3$ | 38920 | 580 | 66.9 |

Peanuts were germinated in presence of glycine-u-$^{14}$C, NaH$^{14}$CO$_3$ and Aspartic-u-$^{14}$C, $10^{-5}$M  L-T$_3$.  RNA was extracted as described in the text.   RNA content of peanut cotyledon tissue at various ages after germination, was calculated on the basis of 1  g  tissue.

TABLE 18

Purine nucleotide composition of RNA in the peanuts.

| Source | Nucleotide | Total cmp | Concentration Total mu moles | Specific activity c pm/mu mole |
|--------|-----------|-----------|------------------------------|-------------------------------|
| Control | AMP | 83.7 | 47 | 1.78 |
| L-T$_3$ | AMP | 248.9 | 46 | 5.41 |
| Control | GMP | 144.8 | 72 | 2.01 |
| L-T$_3$ | GMP | 74.4 | 72 | 1.03 |

Nucleotides were separated by one-dimensional chromatography on Whatman No. 3 MM paper. 0.7 ml of the respective alkaline hydrolyzates were spotted directly. Separations were run at room temperature. Identification of AMP and GMP was described in the text and shown in Table 19. Aliquots of the eluates were transferred to scintillation counting vials, evaporated to dryness, dissolved in hyamine and counted with a Packard Tri-Carb scintillation spectrometer.

## TABLE 19

### Identification of Nucleotides.

| Source | Nucleotide | Rf | Maxima (mu) | | Minima (mu) | | $\frac{250}{260}$ | | $\frac{280}{260}$ | |
|--------|-----------|-----|-----|-----|-----|-----|-----|-----|-----|-----|
| | | | pH7 | pH2 | pH7 | pH2 | pH7 | pH2 | pH7 | pH2 |
| Control | AMP | 0.44 | 258 | 259 | 227 | 228 | .85 | .83 | .13 | .22 |
| L-$T_3$ | AMP | 0.44 | 258 | 259 | 227 | 228 | .81 | .83 | .13 | .22 |
| Authentic | AMP | 0.44 | 258 | 259 | 227 | 230 | .79 | .84 | .15 | .21 |
| Literature | AMP | 0.45 | 259 | 257 | 227 | 230 | .79 | .84 | .15 | .22 |
| Control | GMP | 0.135 | 254 | 257 | 224 | 230 | 1.04 | .96 | .69 | .71 |
| L-$T_3$ | GMP | 0.135 | 254 | 257 | 223 | 230 | 1.09 | .96 | .69 | .70 |
| Authentic | GMP | 0.130 | 252 | 257 | 223 | 229 | 1.16 | .90 | .69 | .68 |
| Literature | GMP | 0.130 | 252 | 257 | 223 | 229. | 1.16 | .90 | .69 | .68 |

The solvent used was system No. I. (isobutyric acid/conc. $NH_4OH$/water, 66%/1/33; ph 3.7). Spots were detected with ultraviolet light, cut out, and eluted with M potassium phosphate buffer pH 7.0 for 18 hours at $37^o$. Identification of these nucleotides was based on Rf, maxima, minima, $\frac{250}{260}$ and $\frac{280}{260}$. Calculation of the nucleotide concentration in the eluates were based on optical density and published extinction data at the respective absorption maxima.

TABLE 20

The effect of triiodo-L-thyronine on protein synthesis in germinating peanuts.

| Addition | $\dfrac{cpm}{mg\ protein}$ |
|---|---|
| None | 526.2 |
| L-T$_3$ | 911.4 |

Peanuts were germinated in presence of glycine-u-$^{14}$C, NaHC$^{14}$O$_3$ and l-Aspartic-u-$^{14}$C with and without L-T$_3$(10$^{-5}$M). Protein was extracted as described in the text. One mg protein of each dried sample was weighed with a Cahn electrobalance, quantitatively transferred to a scintillation counting vial and dissolved in 1.0 ml of M hydroxide of hyamine in methanol by recapping the vials and heating at 60° for approximately one hour. To each vial was added 15 ml of scintillator fluid containing 0.4% PPO and 0.01% POPOP in toluene. Counting was then carried out in a Packard Tri-Carb scintillation counter.

## TABLE 21

Amino acid analysis of the protein in peanuts.

| Amino Acid | Concentration | | C P M | | cpm/ug Specific Activity | |
|---|---|---|---|---|---|---|
| | $+T_3$ | $-T_3$ | $+T_3$ | $-T_3$ | $+T_3$ | $-T_3$ |
| Lysine | 36.6 | 30.3 | 60.5 | 24.5 | 1.65 | .80 |
| Histidine | 27.3 | 23.4 | 30.3 | 26.5 | 1.1 | 1.1 |
| Ammonia | 16.3 | 15.6 | | | | |
| Arginine | 130.6 | 151.1 | 28.2 | 24.0 | .215 | .208 |
| Aspartic | 114.9 | 98.4 | 87.2 | 22.7 | .75 | .231 |
| Threonine | 25.3 | 24.08 | 30.9 | 29.0 | 1.21 | 1.20 |
| Serine | 33.9 | 31.5 | 25.5 | 22.2 | .75 | .70 |
| Glutamic Acid | 178.5 | 150.1 | 116.3 | 16.5 | .65 | .109 |
| Proline | 37.8 | 34.5 | 23.8 | 88 | .62 | .25 |
| Glycine | 37.6 | 34.9 | 15.9 | 28.3 | .42 | .81 |
| Alanine | 40.8 | 27.4 | 46.2 | 28.6 | 1.1 | 1.1 |
| Half cystine | 7.6 | 5.3 | | | | |
| Valine | 51.9 | 46.3 | 49.1 | 46.0 | .94 | 1.0 |
| Methionine | 6.7 | 6.2 | 20 | 15 | 2.9 | 2.4 |
| Isoleucine | 44.2 | 36.7 | 20 | 15 | .45 | .40 |
| Leucine | 68.3 | 61.2 | 25.9 | 22.6 | .38 | .37 |
| Tyrosine | 31.7 | 31.9 | 30.7 | 23.4 | .96 | .73 |
| Phenylalanine | 52.0 | 48.5 | 32.0 | 19.1 | .61 | .39 |
| TOTAL | 942 | 821 | 642.5 | 428.5 | | |

100 mg of soluble protein was hydrolyzed in 10 ml of 6N HCl for 24 hours, The hydrolysate filtered and dried, then dissolved in 40 ml of 0.2 Na citrate buffer pH 2.2 to give a concentration of 1.25 mg/ml and then 1 ml was applied to the column. Amino acid analysis on the column is described in the text.

TABLE  22

Determination of the protein in peanut by the Kjeldahl method.

| Addition | % N | % Protein |
| --- | --- | --- |
| control | 10. 8 | 67. 5 |
| control  L-T$_3$ | 11. 86 | 74. 12 |

Nitrogen analysis were made on the . 35 mg of crude protein isolated from peanut as described in the text.

Fig. 1

Effect of pH on IMP-dehydrogenase. The reaction mixture contained in umoles: NAD, 14.7; IMP, 19.8; Tris-phosphate, 20; total protein 0.4 mg; total volume 1.5 ml. The pH was varied as shown.

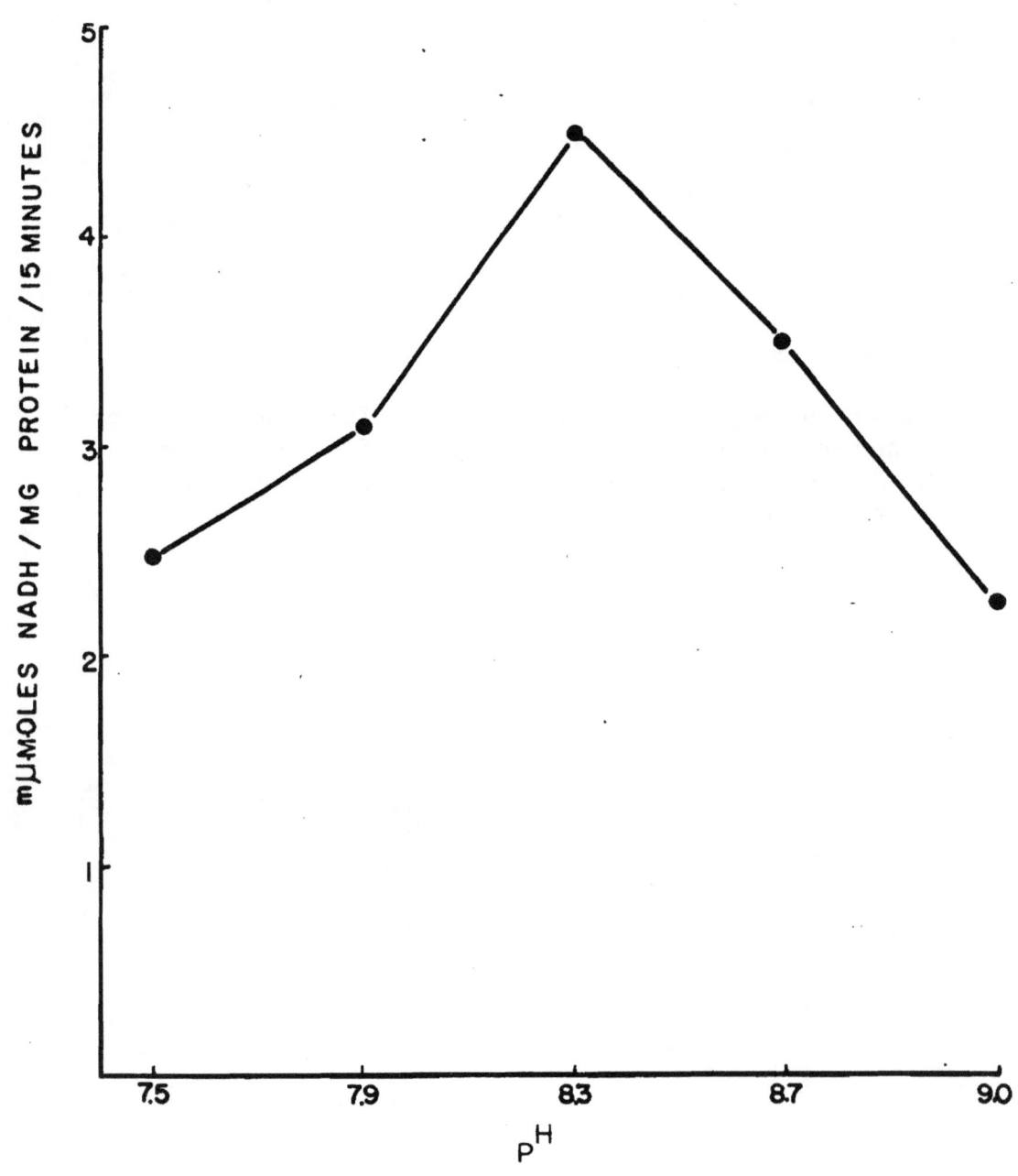

3

Fig. 2

Specificity of IMP-dehydrogenase.  The conditions were as
described in Fig. 1. except NADP when added was 14.7 umole and
protein was 0.25 mg.

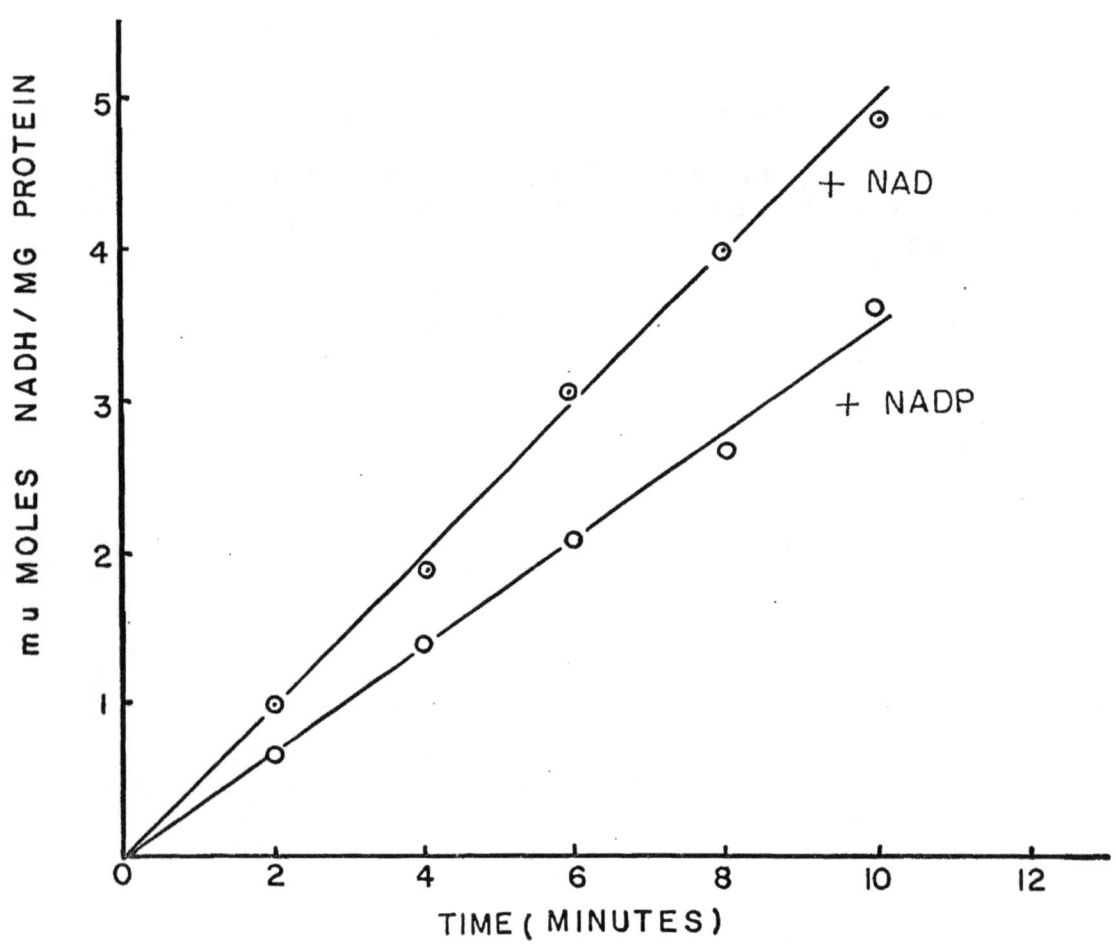

Fig. 3

Inhibition of GMP synthesis by triiodo-L-thyronine.  The
reaction mixture contained in umoles:  NAD, 13; IMP, 20;
glutamine, 100; MgCl$_2$ , 4; Tris-phosphate, pH 7.6, 20; and
60 mg acetone powder.  When added, L-T$_3$ was $10^{-9}$M.  Total
volume was 3.0 ml.  The reaction was stopped by the addition
of 0.2 ml of 3.6 M perchloric acid.  The precipitated protein
was centrifuged out, and absorption at 290 mu was measured
against a blank which contained all ingredients except IMP and
L-T$_3$.

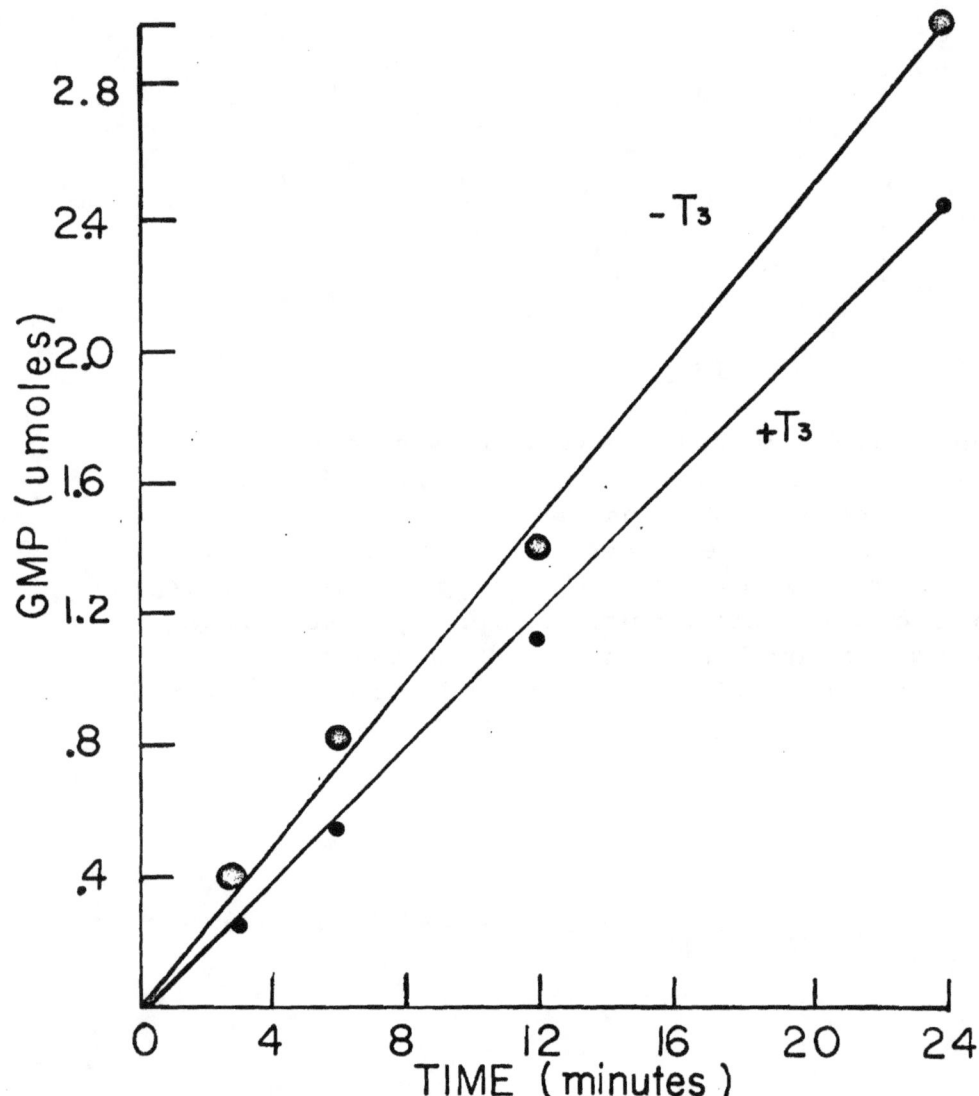

Fig. 4

The inhibition of IMP-dehydrogenase by triiodo-L-thyronine.
Incubation media in umoles: IMP, 19.8; NAD, 14.7; Tris-
phosphate, pH 7.6, 40; and 0.5 ml of the dialyzed supernatant
fraction from 0.14 gm of liver from growth-arrested, sulfaguanidine-fed rat. When added, L-T$_3$ was $10^{-9}$M. Total volume
was 3.0 ml. The change in absorbancy ( $\triangle$ ) was measured
against a blank which contained all ingredients except IMP and
L-T$_3$.

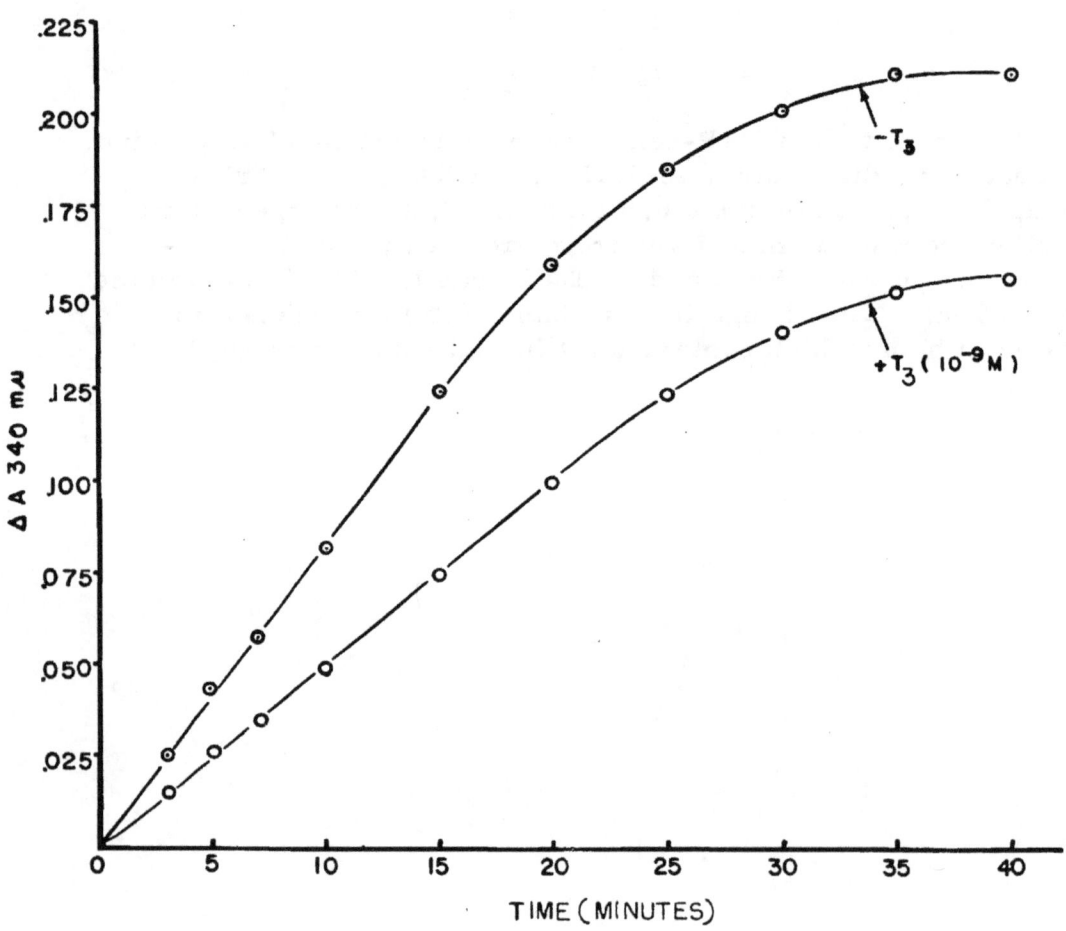

Fig. 5

The effect of Tetraiodo-L-thyronine on IMP dehydrogenase.
The conditions were as described in Table 1. , using the DEAE-
Sephadex treated enzyme and $L-T_4$ was added as indicated. Total
protein: 0.25 mg.

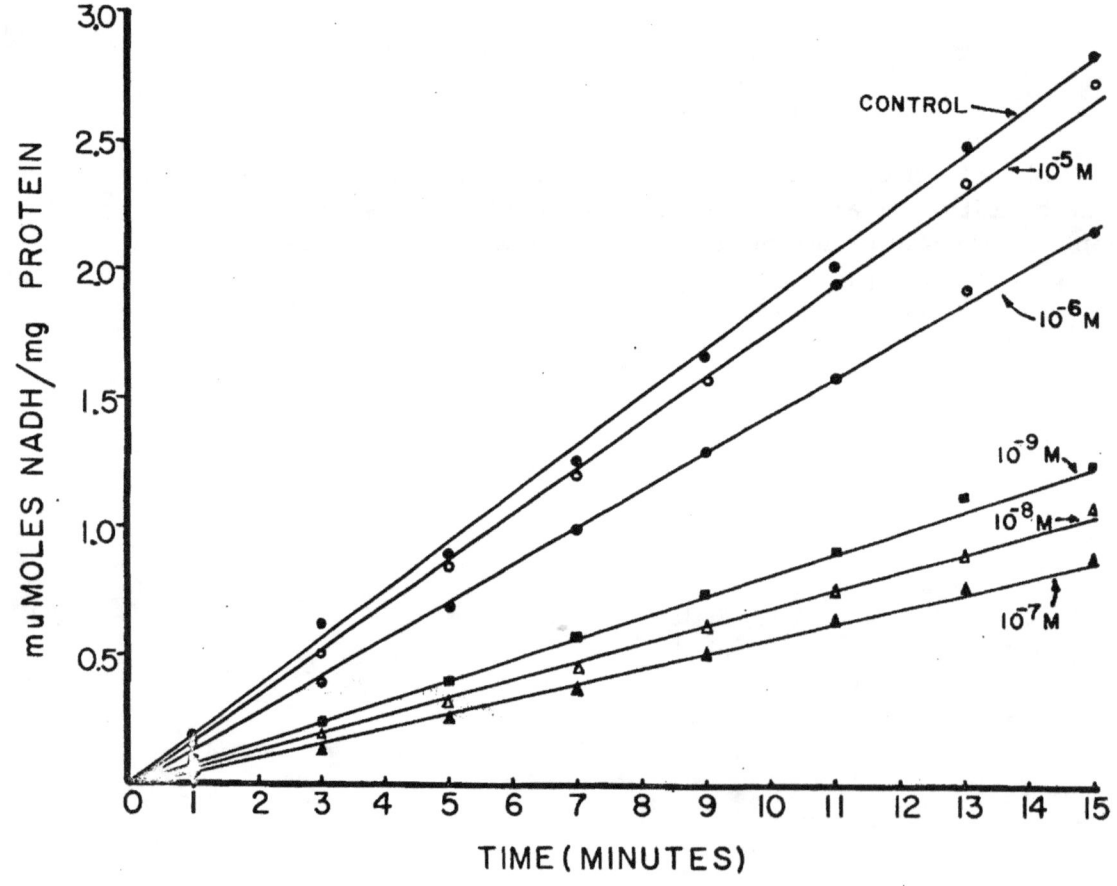

Fig. 6

Optimum concentration of triiodo-L-thyronine. Conditions were as described in Table 1 using the DEAE-Sephadex treated enzyme and the indicated amounts of L-T$_3$. The total protein was 0.3 mg. The results are plotted as a function of hormone concentration to illustrate the maximum inhibition by $10^{-9}$M of triiodo-L-thyronine.

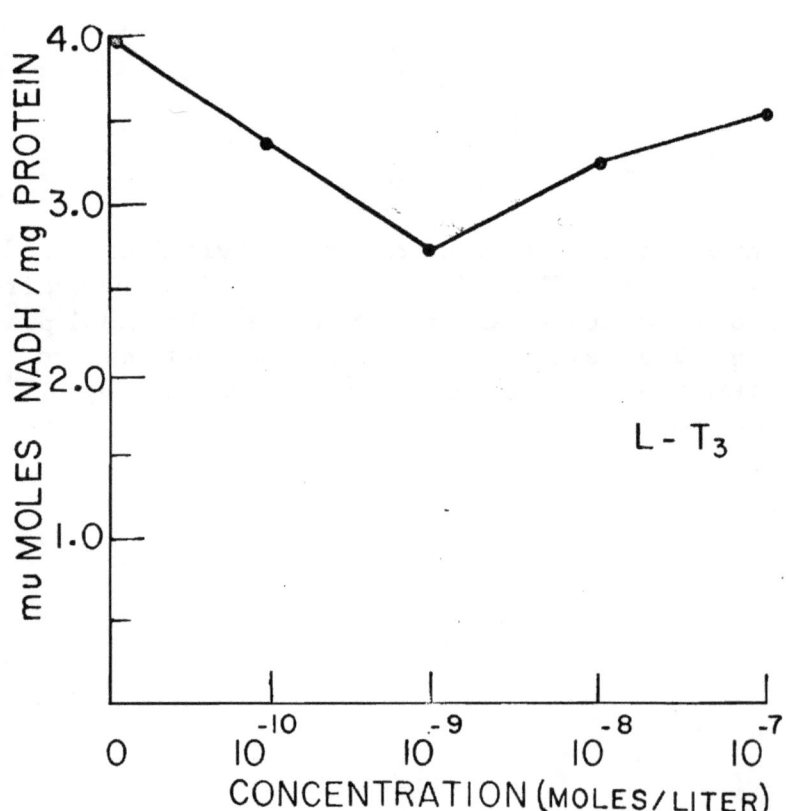

Fig. 7

The effect of tetraiodo-D-thyronine on IMP-dehydrogenase.
Conditions described in Table 1 using the DEAE-Sephadex
treated enzyme except that the indicated amounts of the hormone
were added.  Total protein was 0.24 mg.

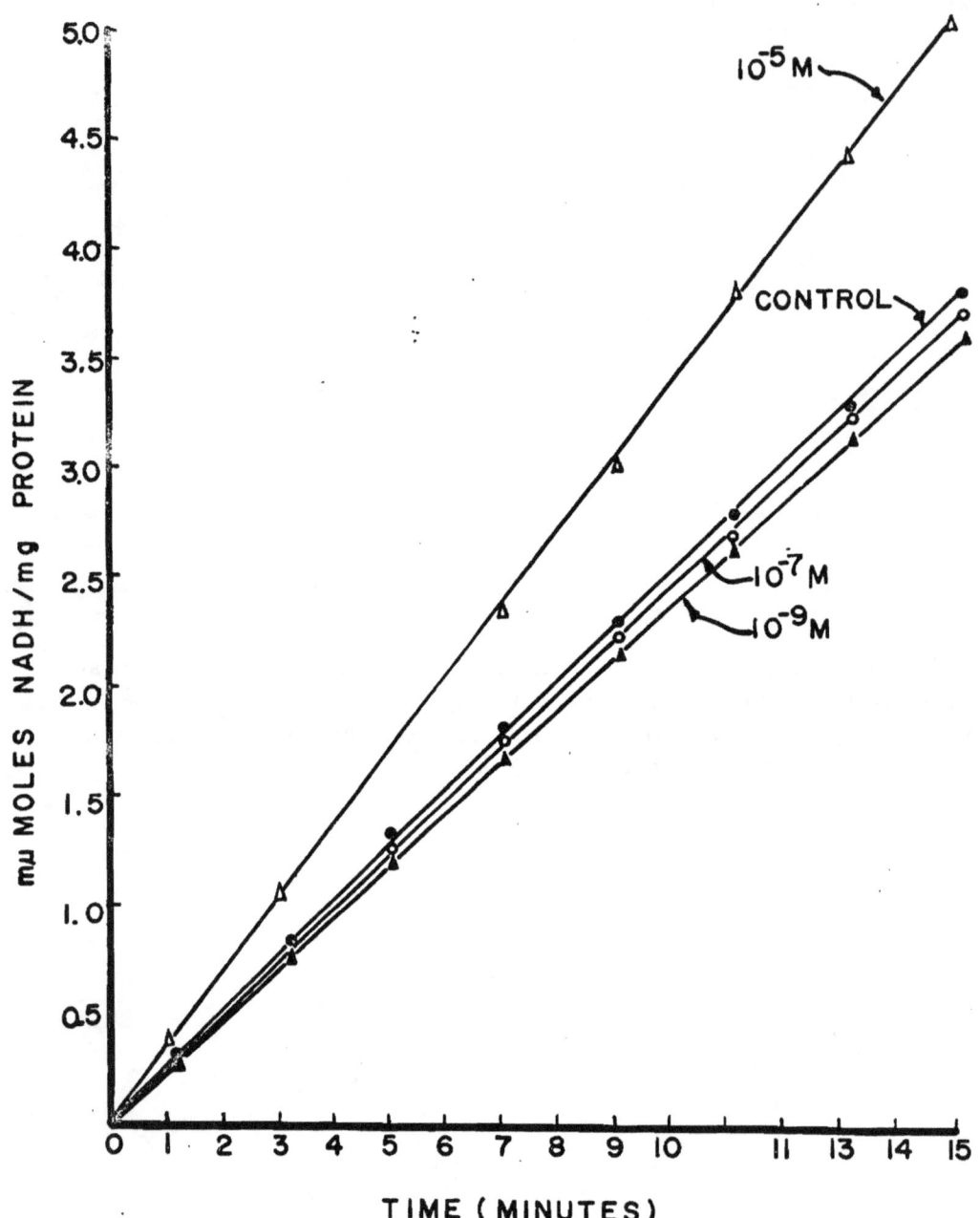

Fig. 8   and Fig. 8a

Inhibition of IMP dehydrogenase by tetraiodo-L-thyronine, triiodo-L-thyronine and a combination of these hormones. Incubation media and procedure were as described under Table 1 using the DEAE-Sephadex treated enzyme.   Total protein was 0.25 mg.

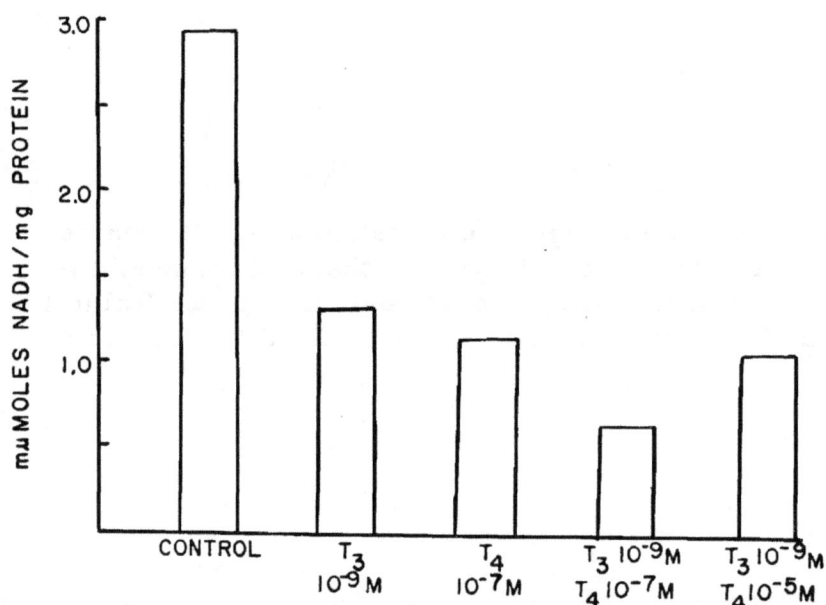

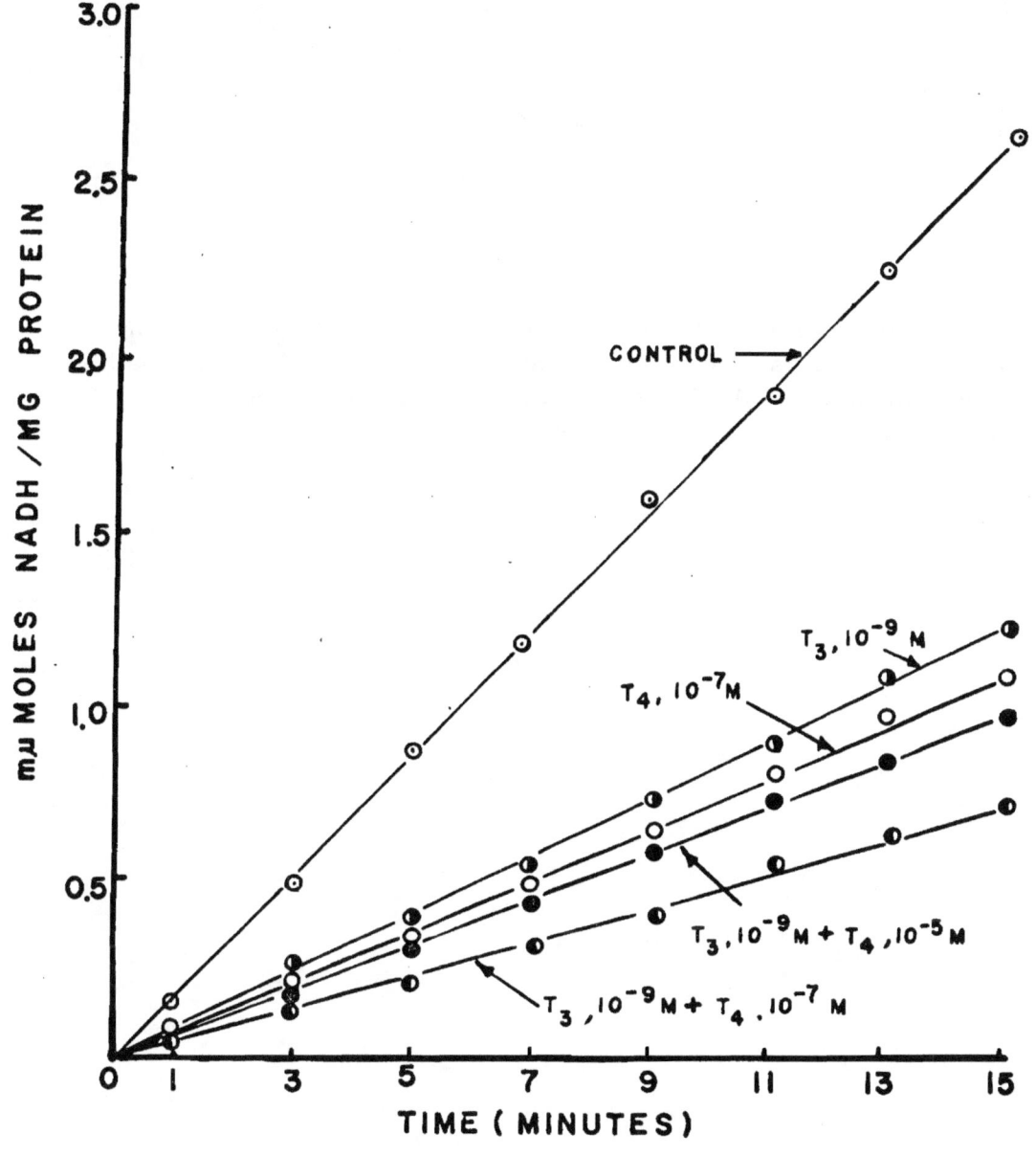

Fig. 9

The effect of 3,5-diiodo-L-tyrosine on IMP dehydrogenase. Conditions were as described in Table 1 using the DEAE-Sephadex treated enzyme and the indicated amounts of the compound were added. Total protein was 0.25 mg.

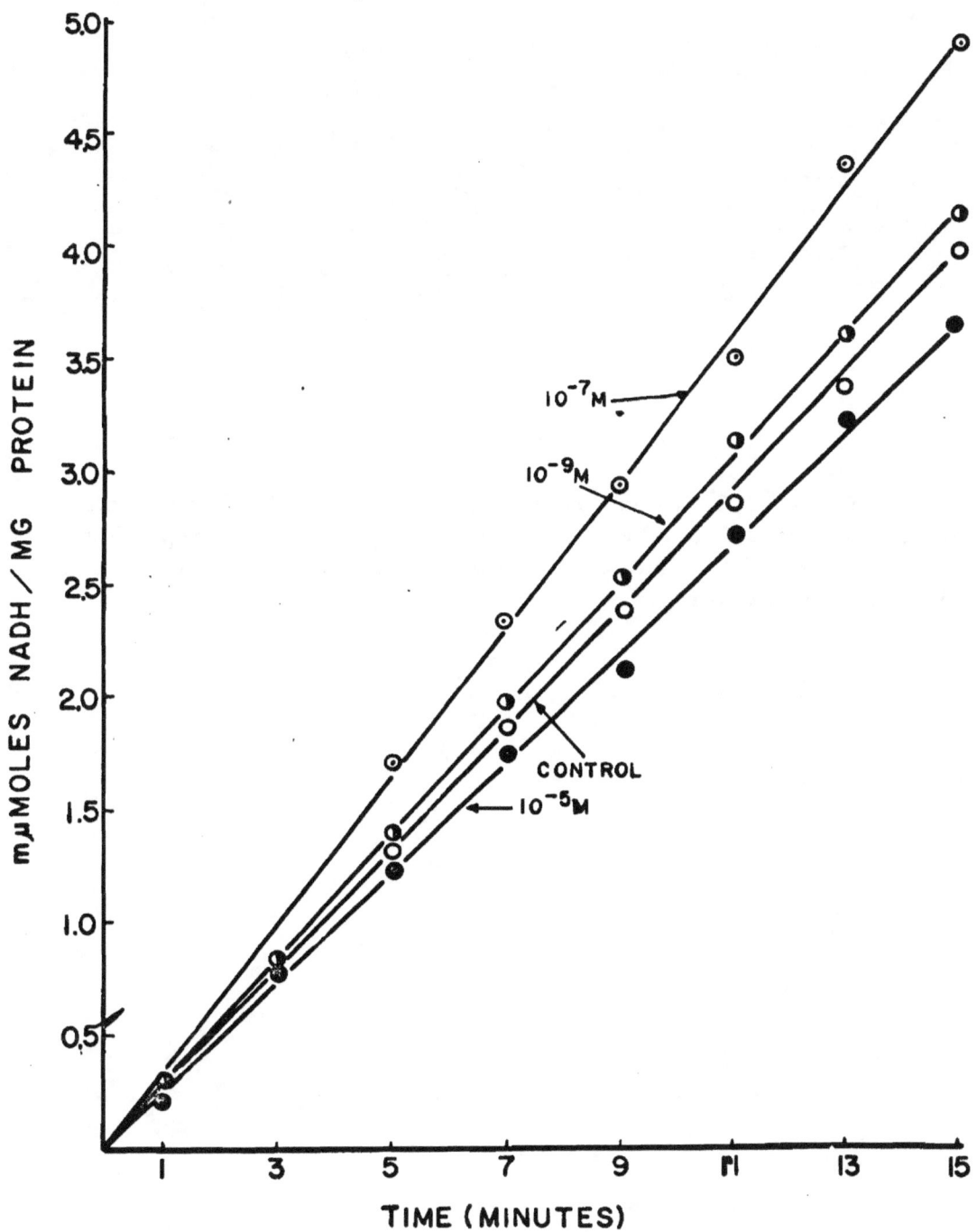

Fig. 10

The effect of 3,5-diiodothyroproprionate on IMP dehydrogenase.
Conditions were as described in Table 1 using the DEAE-Sephadex
treated enzyme and the indicated amount of the analogue was added.
Total protein was 0.8 mg.

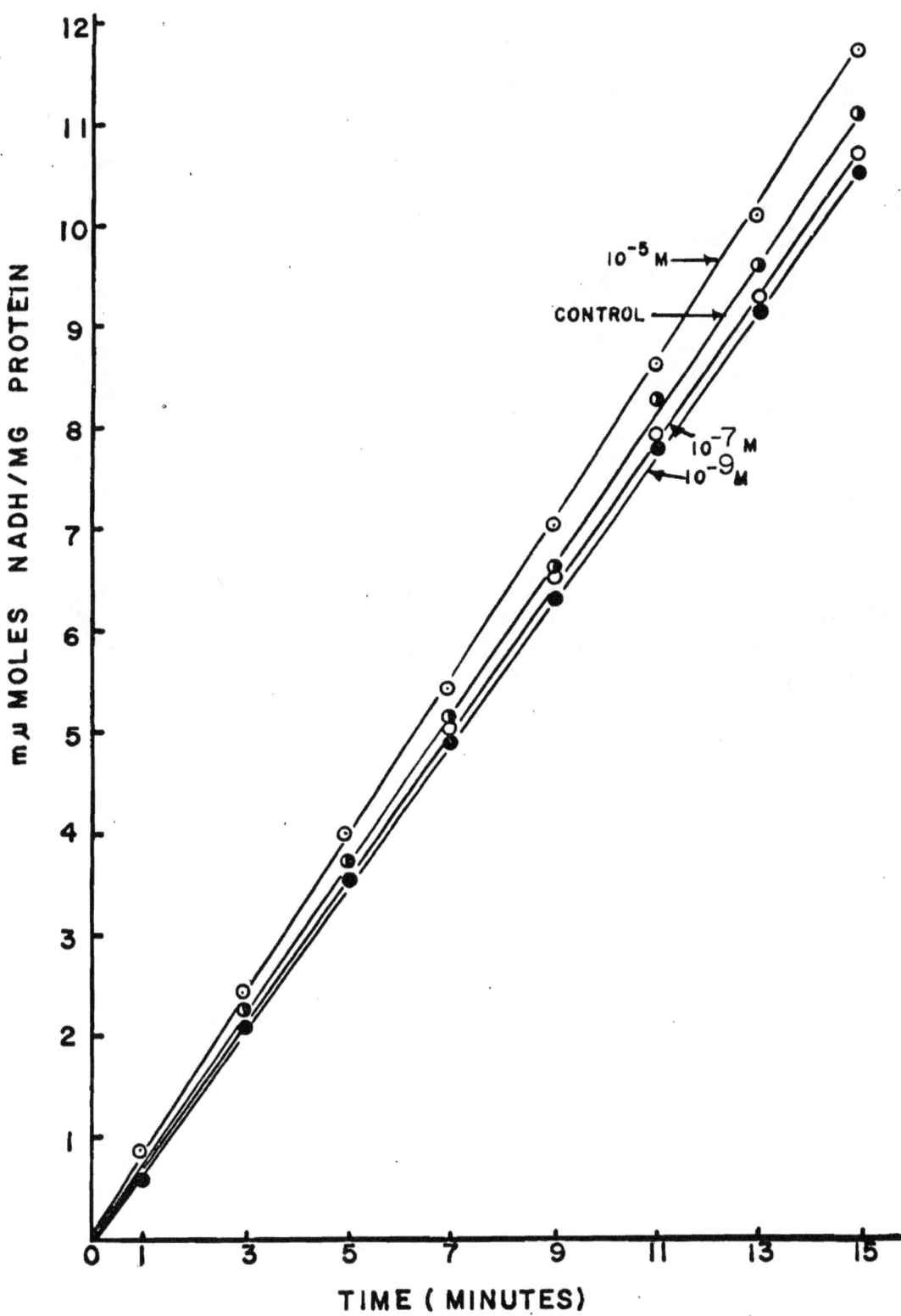

Fig. 11

The effect of 3,5-diiodo-L-thyronine on IMP dehydrogenase. Conditions were described in Table 1 using the DEAE-Sephadex treated enzyme and the indicated amounts of the analogue were added. Total protein was 0.25 mg.

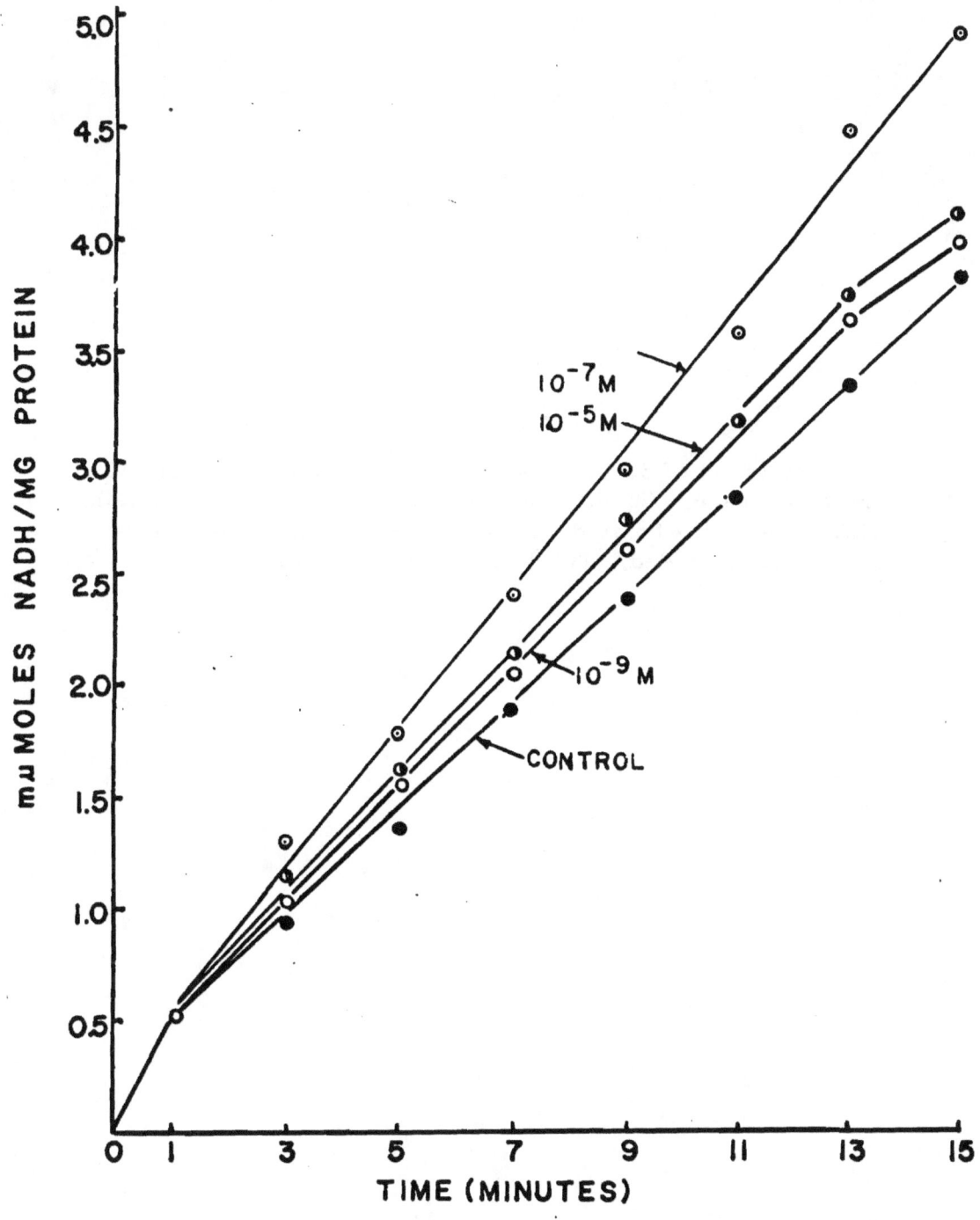

Fig. 12

The effect of 3,5,3',5'-tetraiodothyropropionate on IMP
dehydrogenase.  Conditions are as described in Table 1 using the
DEAE-Sephadex treated enzyme and the indicated amount of the
analogue was added.  Total protein was 0.22 mg.

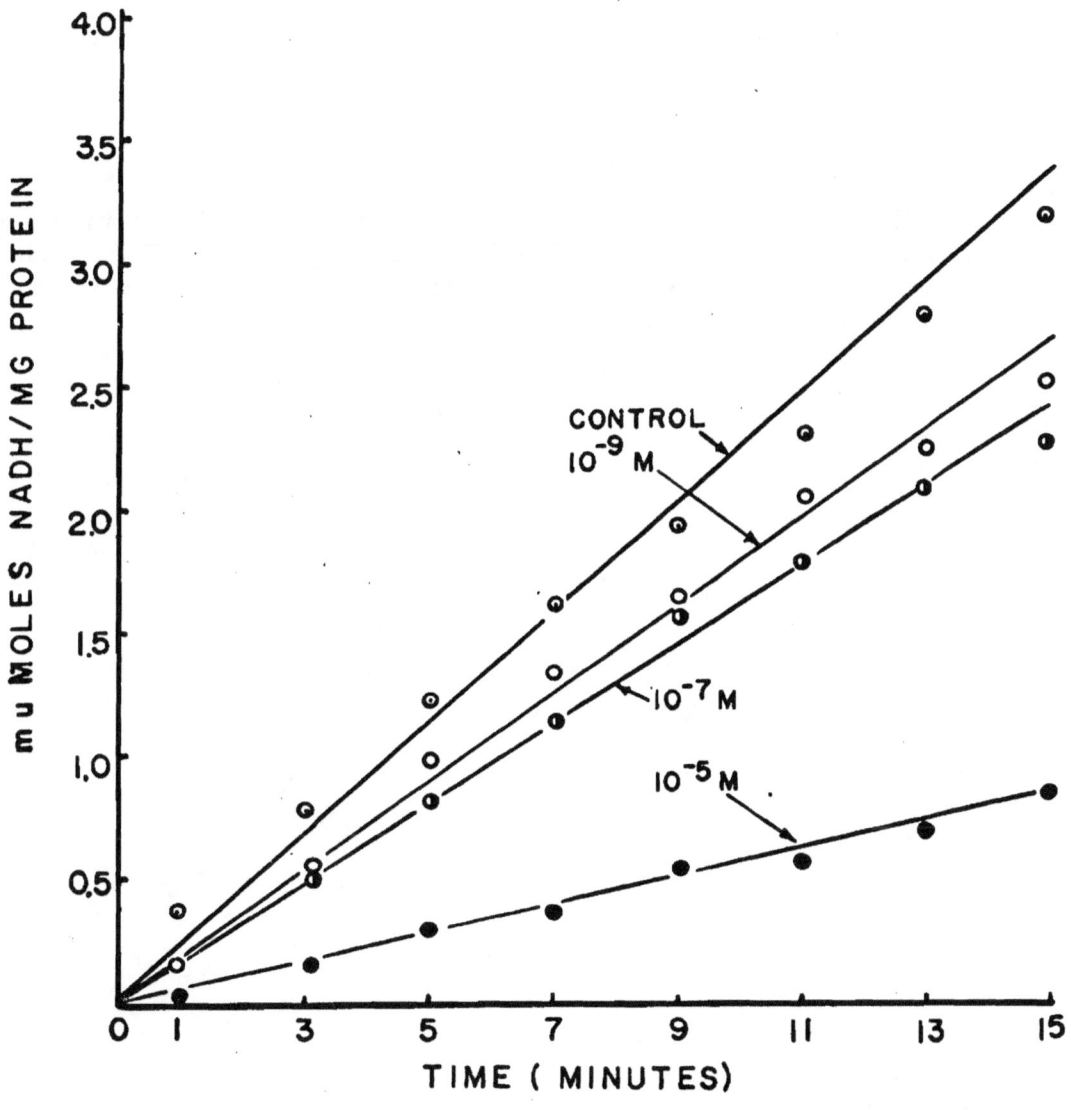

Fig. 13

The effect of 3, 5, 3'-triiodothyropropionate on IMP dehydrogenase. Conditions were as described in Table 1 using the DEAE-Sephadex treated enzyme and the indicated amount of the analogue was added. Total protein was 0.8 mg.

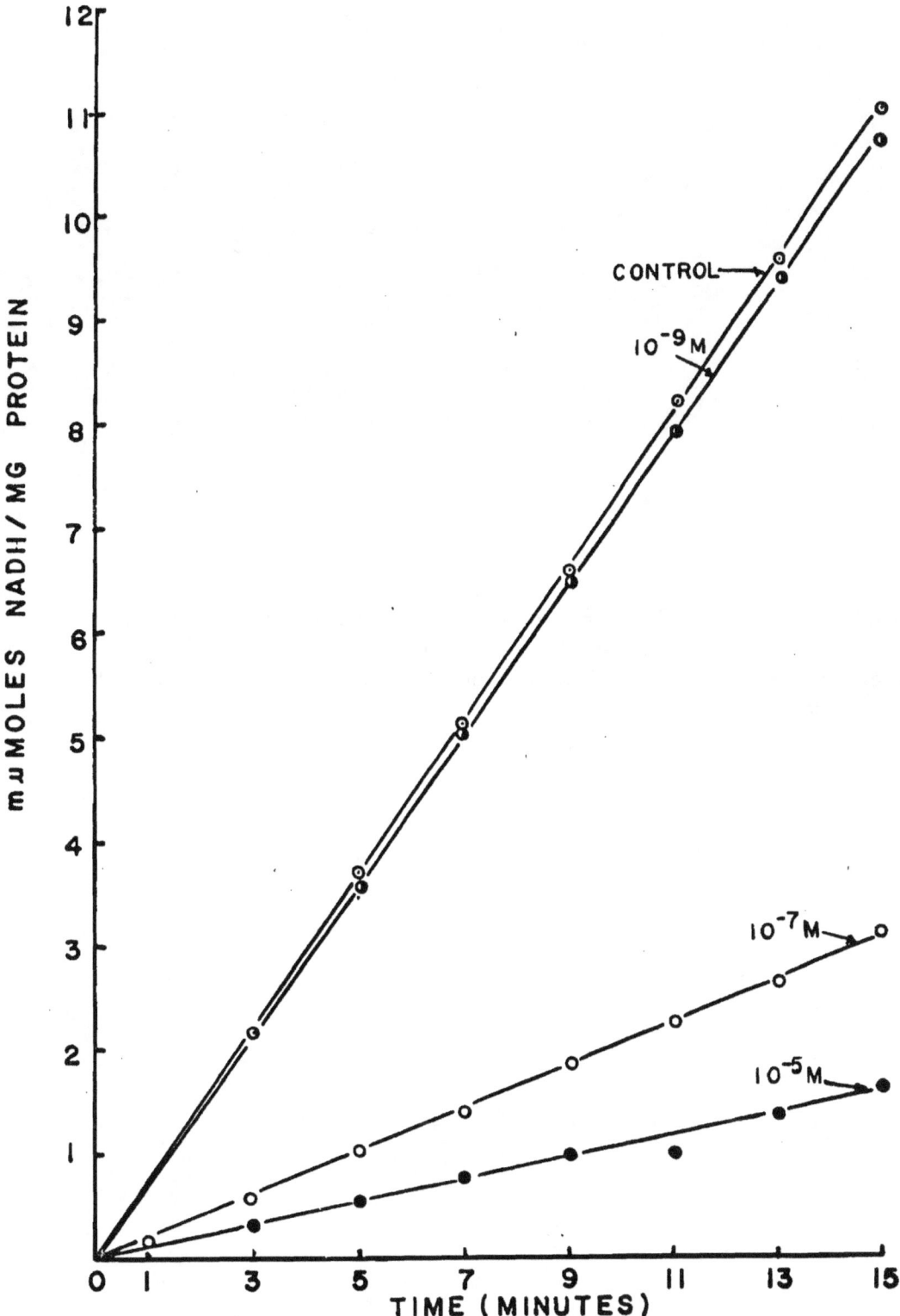

Fig. 14

The effect of 3, 5, 3$'$, 5$'$ -tetraiodo-thyroacetate on IMP dehydrogenase.
Conditions were as described in Table 1 using the DEAE-Sephadex
treated enzyme and the indicated amount of the analogue was added.
Total protein was 0. 23 mg.

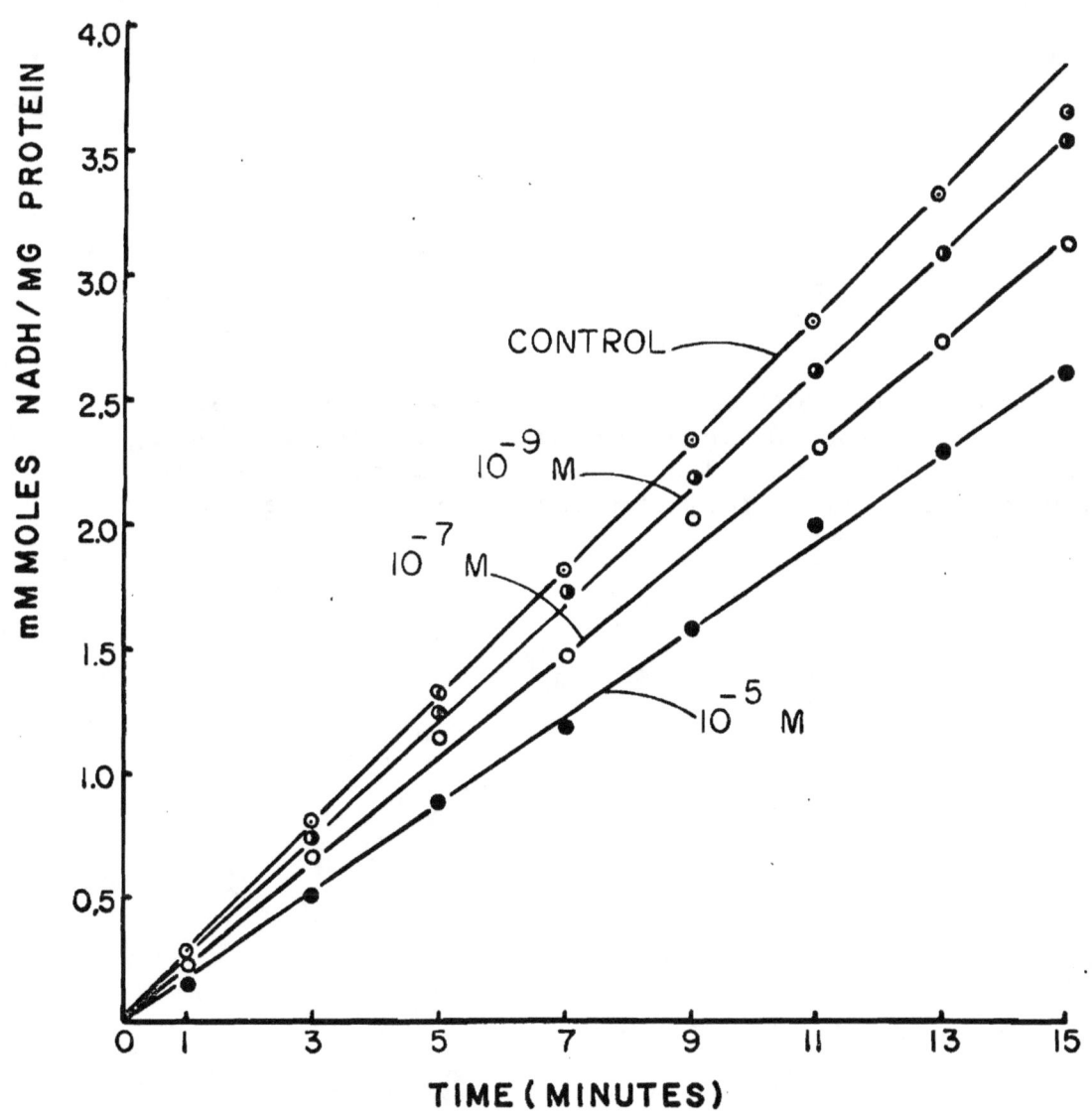

Fig. 15

The effect of thyroid hormones on IMP-dehydrogenase of the
S. Cerevisiae.  The conditions were as described in Table 1 using
the DEAE-Sephadex treated enzyme and the indicated amount of
hormone was added.  Total protein from purified yeast enzyme was
0.30 mg.

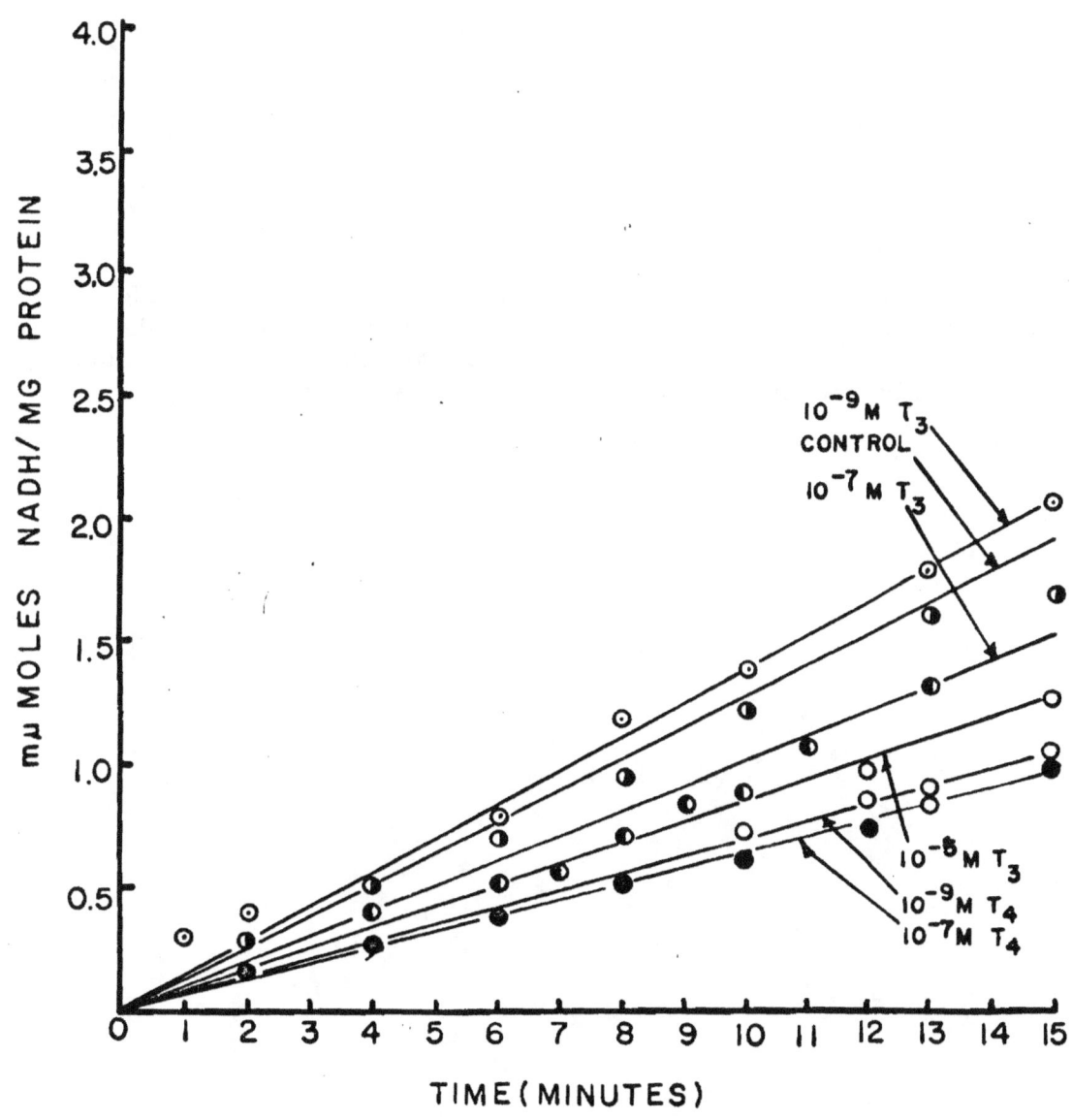

TIME (MINUTES)

Fig. 16

The effect of thyroid hormones on IMP dehydrogenase from Cellvibrio gilvus. Conditions were as described in Table 1 using the DEAE-Sephadex treated enzyme and the indicated amount of the hormones were added. Total protein was 0.32 mg.

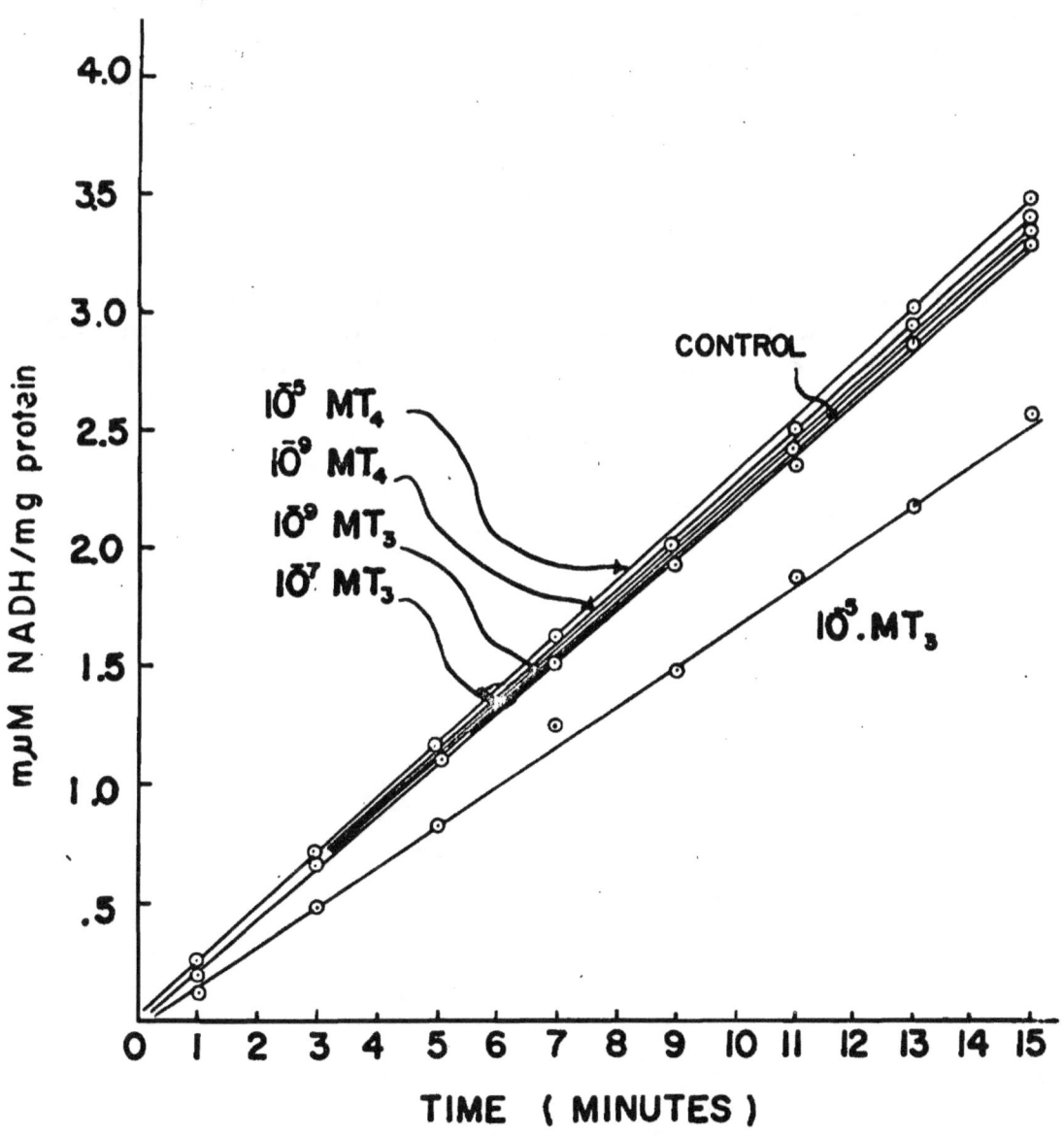

Fig. 17

IMP dehydrogenase from the thorax of American cockroaches.
Conditions are as described in Table 13, except that the enzyme was
purified from thorax of American cockroaches and total protein was
0. 35 mg.

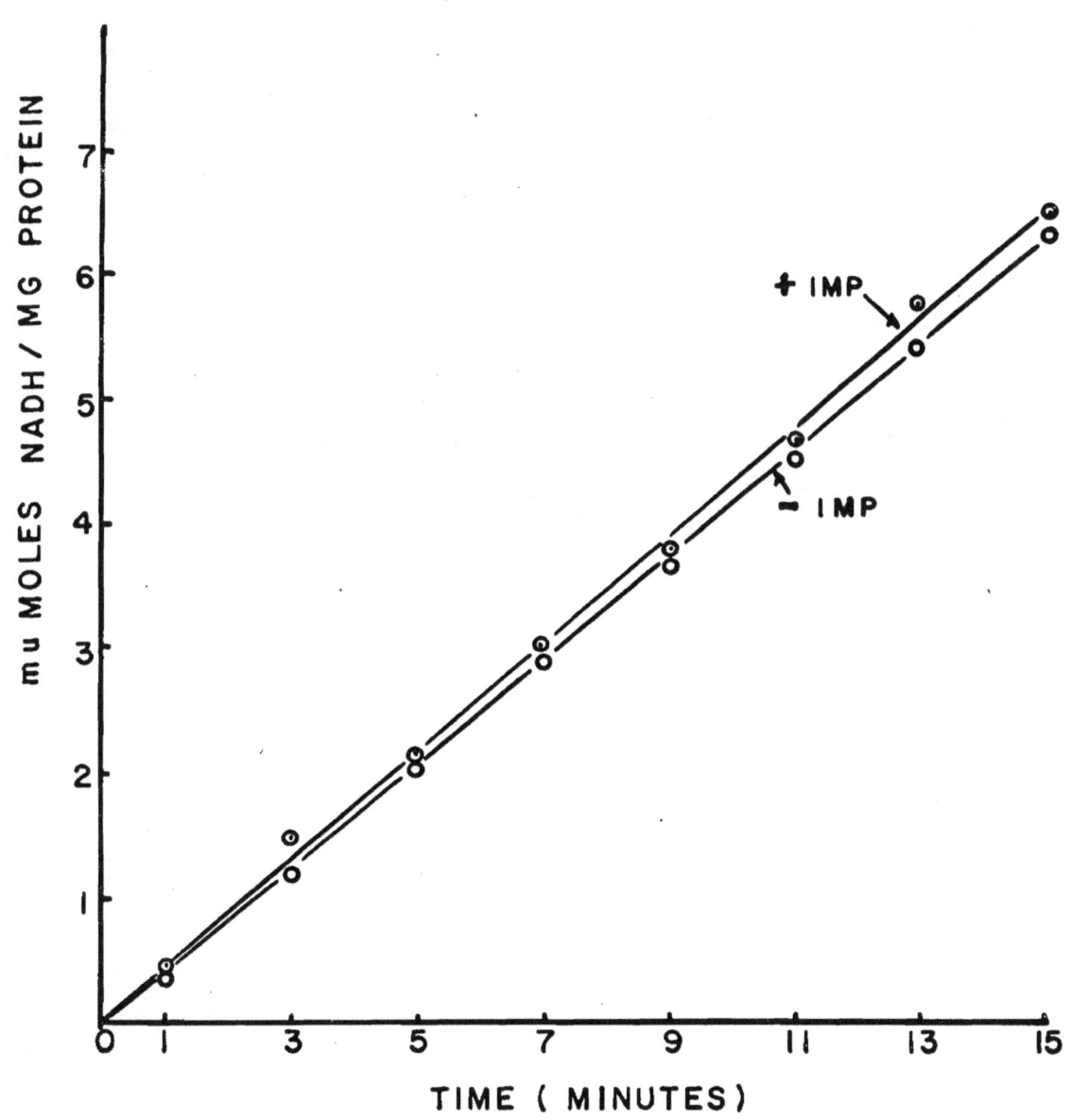

Fig. 18

The effect of thyroid hormones on the growth of American cockroaches. Newly hatched American cockroaches were grown in the presence of thyroid hormones. Conditions as described in the text.

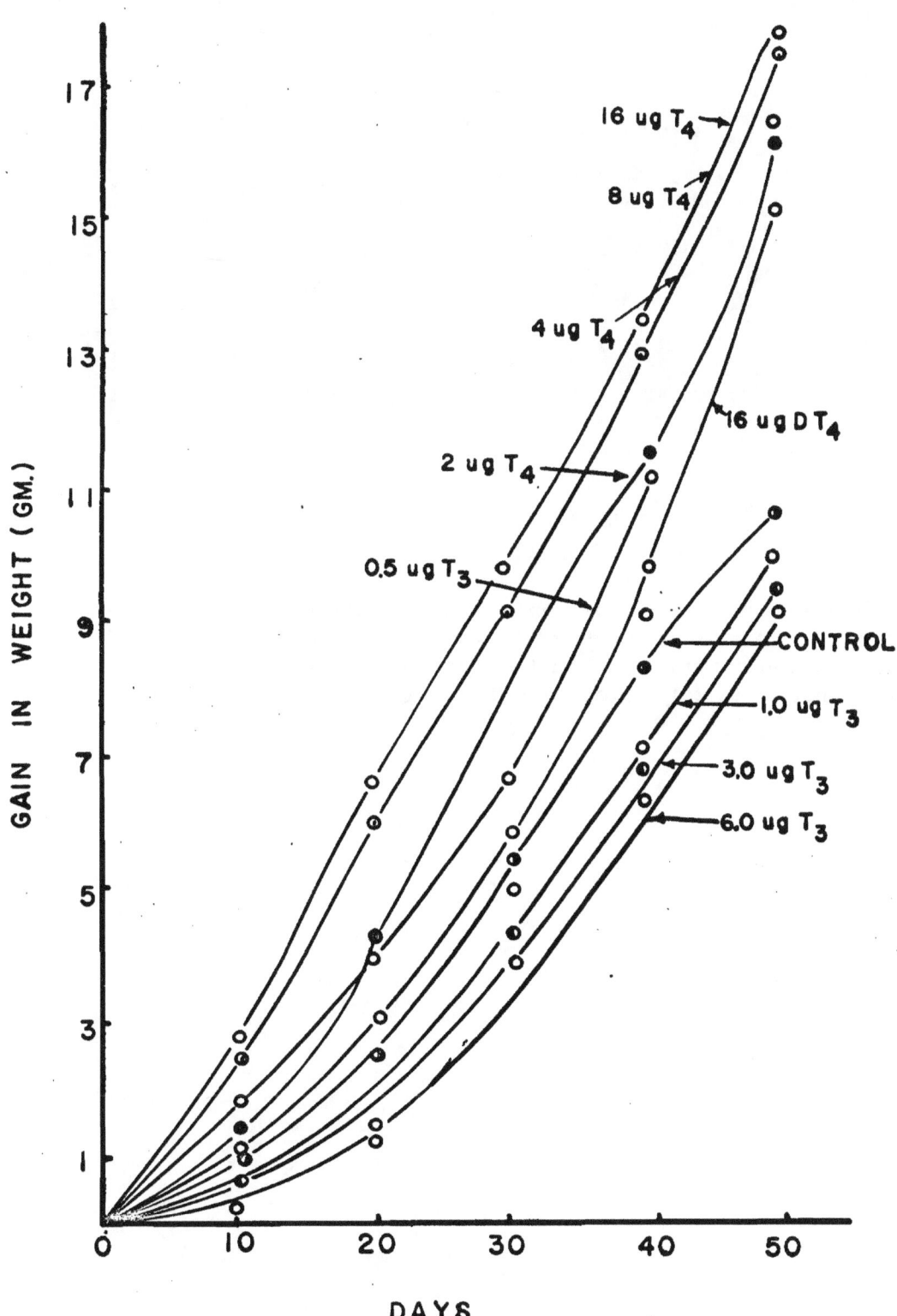

Fig. 19

The effect of thyroid hormones on IMP dehydrogenase abdomen of American cockroaches. Conditions are as described in Table 14, except that the enzyme was purified from abdomen of American cockroaches and total protein was 0.35 mg.

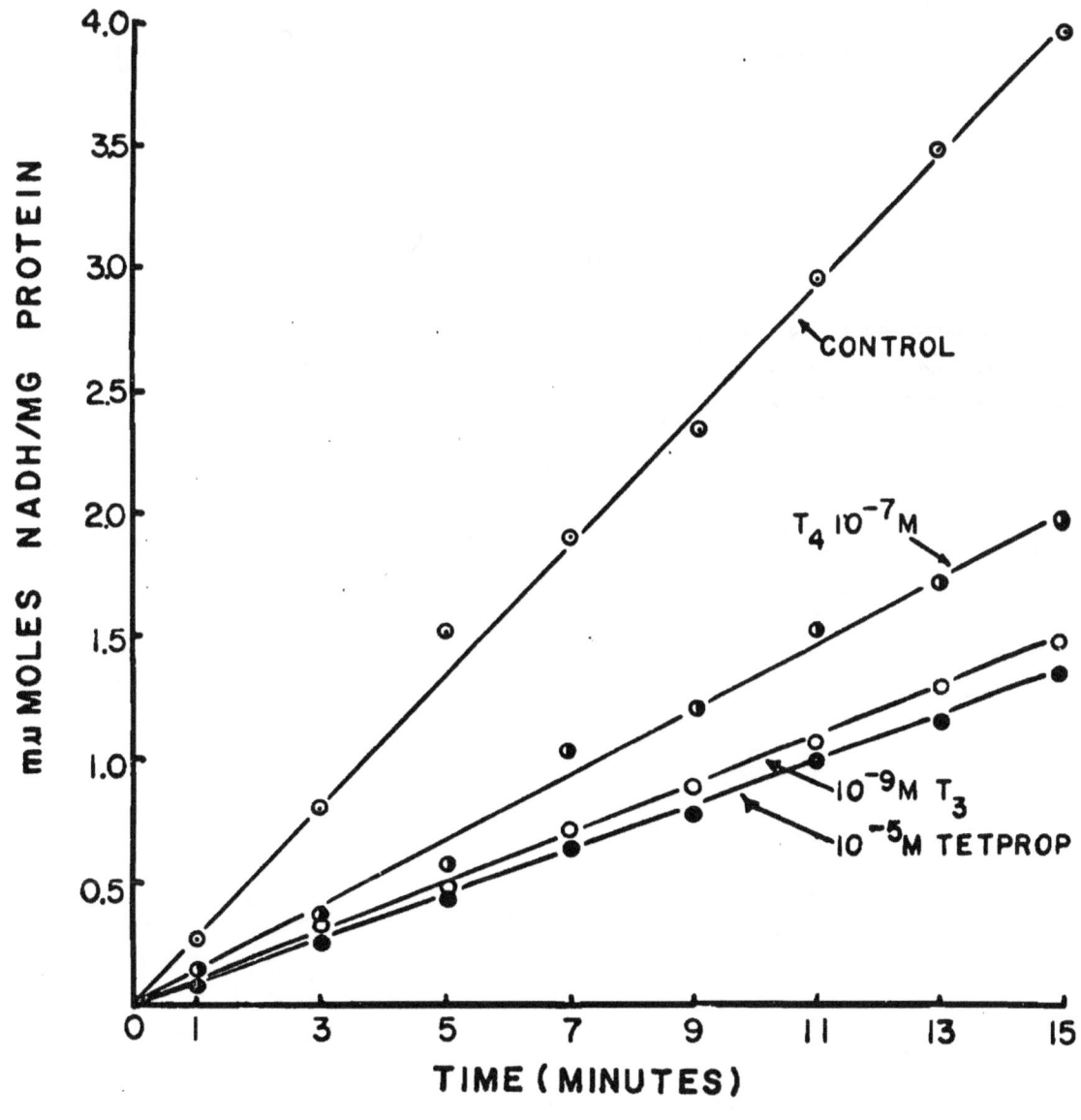

Fig. 20

The effect of thyroid hormones on IMP dehydrogenase of peanuts. Conditions are as described in Table 15, except that the enzyme was purified from peanuts and total protein was 0.38 mg.

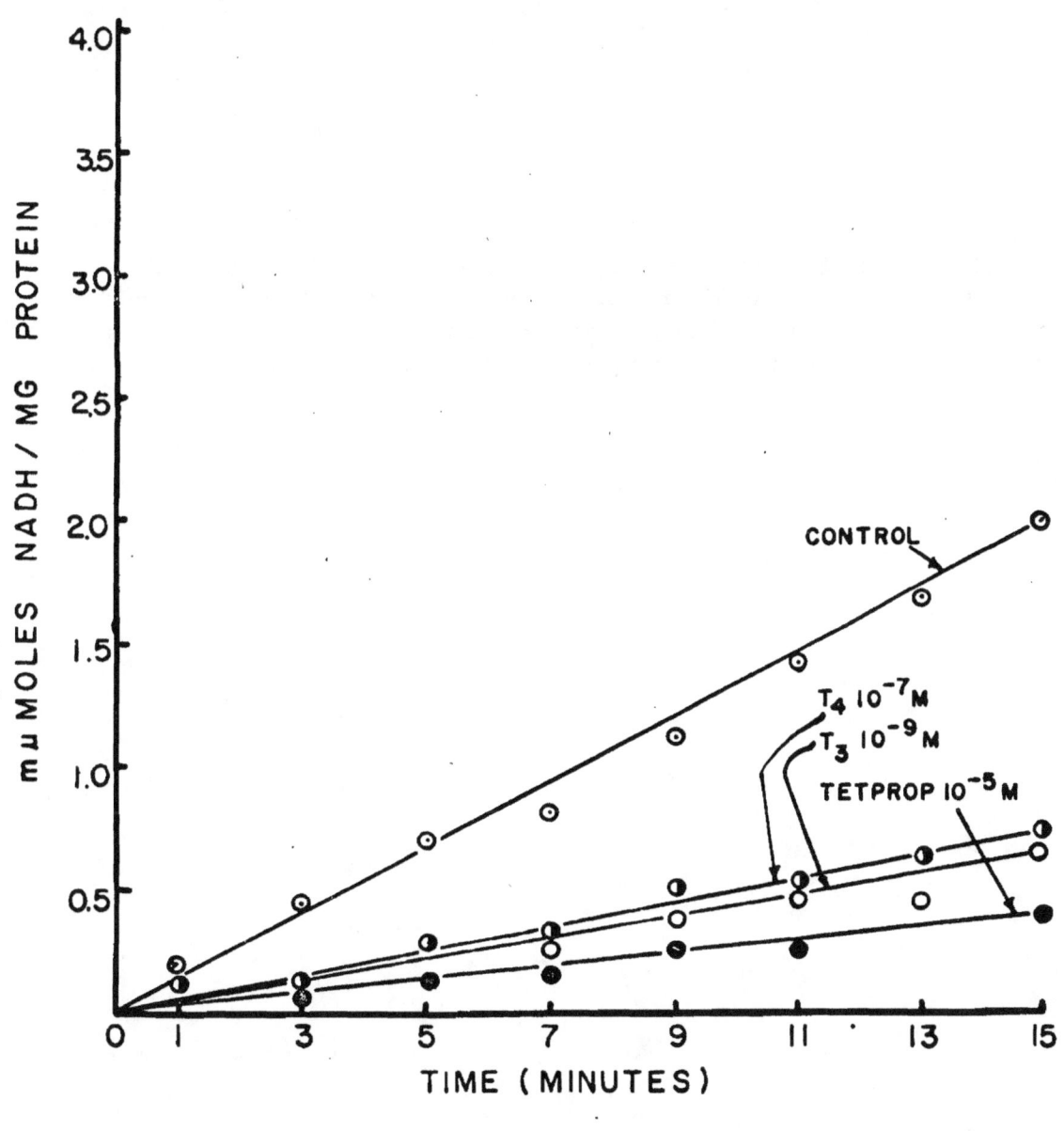

Fig. 21

The effect of thyroid hormones on the growth of peanuts. Ten peanuts were soaked in 100 ml of water or water containing thyroid hormones for 7 hours. They were then transferred to petri plates and allowed to germinate at room temperature in the dark.

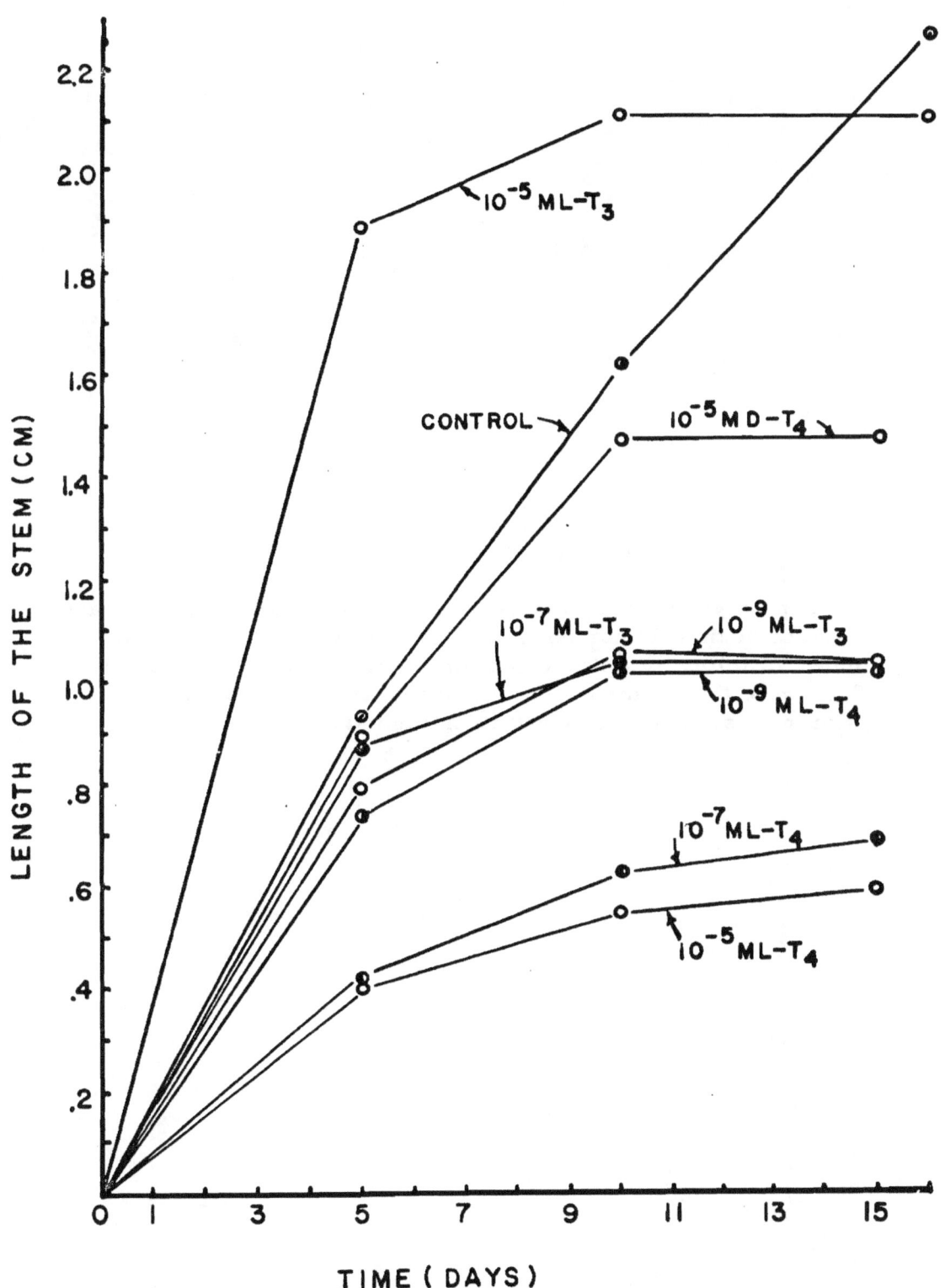

Fig. 22

A photograph of 4 days germinating peanuts in presence and absence of thyroid hormones. Eleven peanuts were soaked in 100 ml of water or water containing thyroid hormones for 7 hours. They were then transferred to petri plates and allowed to germinate at room temperature in the dark.

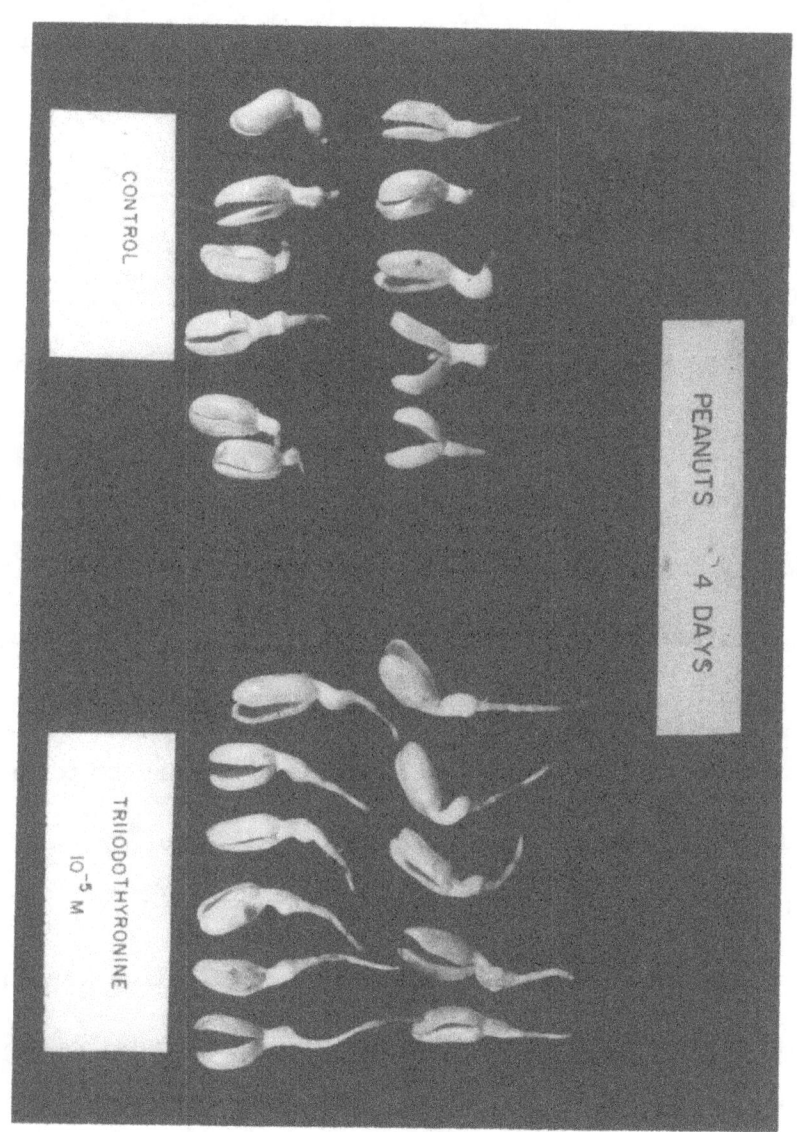

ABSTRACT. STUDIES ON THE MECHANISM OF ACTION OF
THYROID HORMONES by Sami Al-Mudhaffar

Inosine monophosphate (IMP) is a precursor of the two
purine nucleotides, adenosine monophosphate (AMP) and guanosine
monophosphate (GMP): IMP $\longrightarrow$ adenylosuccinate $\longrightarrow$ AMP and
IMP $\longrightarrow$ xanthine monophosphate (XMP) $\longrightarrow$ GMP. The reaction
IMP $\longrightarrow$ adenylosuccinate synthetase which was purified by
$(NH_4)_2 SO_4$ precipitation and by passage through DEAE-Sephadex,
and the reaction IMP $\longrightarrow$ XMP is catalyzed by IMP dehydrogenase
which was purified in a manner similar to adenylosuccinate synthetase.
Adenylosuccinate synthetase of rat liver is stimulated maximally
with $10^{-9}$ M  L-$T_3$ or $10^{-5}$ M  L-$T_4$, but not by D-$T_4$, and the effect
of other analogues paralleled their in vivo effects.  The enzyme,
IMP dehydrogenase, is inhibited by thyroid hormones, but not by
D-$T_4$, and also, the effects of other analogues paralleled their
in vivo effects.  Further correlation to in vivo studies was obtained
from brain and testes tissues.  AMP and GMP synthesis were not
affected by thyroid hormones.  The very low effective concentration
of the hormones on these enzymes, the ineffectiveness of physiologically
inactive thyronine derivatives, the ineffectiveness of these
hormones on these enzymes from brain and testes, and the

importance of these enzymes to energy and nucleic acid metabolism fits the concept of a site of action for thyroid hormones better than many previous suggestions.

These results form the basis of a hypothesis in which thyroid hormones control the energy (ATP) level of the cell and control the synthesis of nucleic acids in the nucleus. A model system to study this was needed and so various organisms were tested for their response to thyroid hormones. Yeast, cockroaches, and peanuts were stimulated (growth) by thyroid hormones. The two enzymes were isolated from these organisms and their response to thyroid hormones tested. The two enzymes from peanuts behaved in a manner similar to the rat enzymes. When peanuts were grown in the presence of thyroid hormones, the specific activity of AMP and GMP was such that is supported the theory that AMP should be high and GMP should be low. It is planned to consider further the use of peanuts as a model system and to investigate the effect of thyroid hormones on the synthesis of RNA and protein in the nucleus.